Mindfulness-Based Interventions for Trauma and Its Consequences

Concise Guides on Trauma Care Series

Mindfulness-Based Interventions for Trauma and Its Consequences

David J. Kearney
Tracy L. Simpson

AMERICAN PSYCHOLOGICAL ASSOCIATION
Washington, DC

The opinions and statements published are the responsibility of the authors, and such opinions and statements do not necessarily represent the policies of the American Psychological Association.

This material is the result of work supported with resources and the use of facilities at VA Puget Sound Health Care System. The contents do not represent the views of the U.S. Department of Veterans Affairs or the United States Government.

Published by
American Psychological Association
750 First Street, NE
Washington, DC 20002
https://www.apa.org

Order Department
https://www.apa.org/pubs/books
order@apa.org

In the U.K., Europe, Africa, and the Middle East, copies may be ordered from Eurospan
https://www.eurospanbookstore.com/apa
info@eurospangroup.com

Typeset in Charter and Interstate by Circle Graphics, Inc., Reisterstown, MD

Printer: Sheridan Books, Chelsea, MI
Cover Designer: Mercury Publishing Services, Inc., Rockville, MD, from an image created by Tracy L. Simpson

Library of Congress Cataloging-in-Publication Data

Names: Kearney, David J., author. | Simpson, Tracy L. (Tracy Lynn), author. |
   American Psychological Association, issuing body.
Title: Mindfulness-based interventions for trauma and its consequences /
   David J. Kearney and Tracy L. Simpson.
Description: Washington, DC : American Psychological Association, [2020] |
   Series: Concise guides on trauma care series | Includes bibliographical
   references and index.
Identifiers: LCCN 2019011708 (print) | LCCN 2019013014 (ebook) |
   ISBN 9781433831447 (eBook) | ISBN 1433831449 (eBook) |
   ISBN 9781433830617 (pbk.) | ISBN 1433830612 (pbk.)
Subjects: | MESH: Stress Disorders, Post-Traumatic—therapy | Psychological
   Trauma—therapy | Mindfulness—methods
Classification: LCC RC552.P67 (ebook) | LCC RC552.P67 (print) | NLM WM 172.5 |
   DDC 616.85/21—dc23
LC record available at https://lccn.loc.gov/2019011708

http://dx.doi.org/10.1037/0000154-000

Printed in the United States of America

10 9 8 7 6 5 4 3 2 1

Contents

Series Foreword

Exposure to traumatic events is all too common, increasing the risk for a range of significant mental problems, such as posttraumatic stress disorder (PTSD) and depression; physical health problems; negative health behaviors, such as smoking and excessive alcohol consumption; impaired social and occupational functioning; and overall lower quality of life. As mass traumas (e.g., September 11th, military engagements in Iraq and Afghanistan, natural disasters such as Hurricane Katrina) have propelled trauma into a brighter public spotlight, the number of trauma survivors seeking services for mental health consequences will likely increase. Yet despite the far-ranging consequences of trauma and the high rates of exposure, relatively little emphasis is placed on trauma education in undergraduate and graduate training programs for mental health service providers in the United States. Calls for action have appeared in the American Psychological Association's journal *Psychological Trauma: Theory, Research, Practice, and Policy* with such articles as "The Need for Inclusion of Psychological Trauma in the Professional Curriculum: A Call to Action," by Christine A. Courtois and Steven N. Gold (2009); and "The Art and Science of Trauma-Focused Training and Education," by Anne P. DePrince and Elana Newman (2011). The lack of education in the assessment and treatment of trauma-related distress and associated clinical issues at undergraduate and graduate levels increases the urgency to develop effective trauma resources for students as well as postgraduate professionals.

This book series, Concise Guides on Trauma Care, addresses that urgent need by providing truly translational books that bring the best of trauma psychology science to mental health professions working in diverse settings. To do so, the series focuses on what we know (and do not know) about specific trauma topics, with attention to how trauma psychology science translates to diverse populations (diversity broadly defined, in terms of development, ethnicity, socioeconomic status, sexual orientation, and so forth).

This series represents one of many efforts undertaken by Division 56 (Trauma Psychology) of the American Psychological Association to advance trauma training and education (https://www.apatraumadivision.org/68/teaching-training.html). We are pleased to work with Division 56 and a volunteer editorial board to develop this series, which continues to move forward with the publication of this important guide on mindfulness-based interventions for trauma by David J. Kearney and Tracy L. Simpson. As clinicians, researchers, and policy makers seek to better understand the effectiveness of interventions for individuals suffering from the consequences of trauma exposure, this monograph offers a practical and accessible guide on mindfulness-based interventions. The authors' discussion on the empirical literature and clinical considerations regarding mindfulness practices will be of great use to mental health professionals when working with individuals suffering from a range of trauma-related symptoms including post-traumatic stress, depression, substance misuse, chronic pain, and other somatic syndromes. Future books in the series will continue to address a range of assessment, treatment, and developmental issues in trauma-informed care.

Ann T. Chu
Anne P. DePrince
Series Editors

Mindfulness-Based Interventions for Trauma and Its Consequences

INTRODUCTION

Our journey teaching, researching, and organizing mindfulness programs did not begin with a focus on trauma or posttraumatic stress disorder (PTSD). Instead, my (David Kearney's) aim nearly 15 years ago was to offer mindfulness programs with the hope that teaching mindfulness would mitigate the suffering of patients with chronic medical conditions. Although the system in which I practice medicine, a large academic Department of Veterans Affairs (VA) hospital, was adept at providing state-of-the art testing and an up-to-date array of medications, surgeries, and procedures to treat symptoms and ailments, what seemed needed were more avenues to help people take a more active role in caring for themselves, especially when faced with difficulties that could not be cured or made to go away.

I had been introduced to meditation practice in the 1980s as a medical student, when I sat in on a group led by some ahead-of-their-time therapists who encouraged people with substance use disorders to meditate. I recall at the time being immediately struck by how setting aside a few minutes each day for meditation practice helped me to maintain a sense of centeredness throughout the day, and how the practice felt intuitively healthy and

http://dx.doi.org/10.1037/0000154-001
Mindfulness-Based Interventions for Trauma and Its Consequences, by D. J. Kearney and T. L. Simpson

important. From that point forward, over many years, I attempted to gradually educate myself about meditation practice in parallel with my efforts to continually deepen my knowledge of the practice of medicine and my specialty of gastroenterology.

Over the course of several years practicing as a physician, as I listened to patients talk of their symptoms, their worries, and their difficulties, I began to wonder why we were not teaching mindfulness. Teaching mindfulness to people with medical problems seemed logical and important, given not just my personal understanding but also knowledge gleaned from the research literature that psychological factors, including daily life stress, fear of symptoms, catastrophizing and beliefs about the meaning of symptoms often worsened conditions such as irritable bowel syndrome and chronic pain. As a clinician I sensed an unmet need for patients, and as a researcher I noted gaps in the scientific literature I could help to fill. With these goals in mind I established a mindfulness program in our hospital and set about coleading, alongside an experienced mindfulness teacher, the initial mindfulness groups for people with medical conditions such as chronic pain and irritable bowel syndrome (IBS).

What I did not expect were the frequent comments by participants about how mindfulness practices seemed to help their symptoms of PTSD. In fact, many patients with PTSD have reported to us that they found the 8-week mindfulness course to be among the most helpful interventions in which they had participated. It is also not uncommon for individuals with PTSD to take the course multiple times so that they can learn more about mindfulness with the support of a group and a teacher. The mindfulness programs at our site gradually expanded to two campuses of a hospital system that serves a population of over 100,000 veterans with a high prevalence of trauma, PTSD, depression, chronic pain and substance misuse. At the time we started offering mindfulness-based stress reduction (MBSR), reports of outcomes for people with PTSD had not yet been published. Given the profound impact of PTSD on individuals across the lifespan, investigating these unexpected reports of benefit for PTSD became a primary focus, and it led to a partnership with Dr. Simpson to further investigate the impact of mindfulness on PTSD.

In many ways my (Tracy Simpson) journey to investigating the potential of mindfulness practice for treating psychological disorders, such as PTSD and their common physical comorbidities, parallels that of Dr. Kearney's. As a clinical psychology graduate student, I initiated a personal meditation practice in an effort to cope with the pressures and stress associated with graduate training and the attendant weight of responsibility I felt being a novice therapist to people with significant distress. Formal meditation time became something of an emotional sanctuary that allowed me to ease up on my expectations of myself and to be more patient with others; generally, it was a quality-of-life saver. I did not yet, however, have the tools needed to bring what I was learning on my own into my clinical work and specifically chose to take a postdoctoral position in the late Dr. Alan Marlatt's lab at the University of Washington to gain exposure to therapeutic applications of mindfulness practices in the addiction realm, my general area of inquiry. From there I transitioned to the Seattle VA and directed the then Women's PTSD Outpatient Clinic. I had the good fortune to begin working with Dr. Kearney at the Seattle VA on formally evaluating whether courses in mindfulness meditation practices could address the psychological, emotional, and social challenges, including PTSD and chronic stress-related physical conditions, that our veteran patients were bringing into our clinics daily.

Together, our interdisciplinary work has sought to understand how mindfulness-based interventions (MBIs) influence conditions commonly borne by people with trauma. Over the past decade we have facilitated thousands of clinical encounters teaching mindfulness to individuals with a history of trauma and enrolled several hundred individuals with PTSD in quantitative and qualitative research studies. Much of the material in this book is based on sharing this extensive clinical and research experience, along with an effort to summarize and make sense of the broader research literature on this topic. From a clinical perspective, what became clear is that given the multiplicity of clinical challenges faced by many people with a history of trauma, an optimal treatment strategy would not only address symptoms of PTSD and depression but also favorably impact physical health problems that commonly co-occur (e.g., chronic pain; Kearney & Simpson, 2015). What can be considered a common factor for many people with these overlapping conditions are experiences of trauma, which can lead to a host of life challenges.

Most people experience traumatic events over the course of their lives. The majority recover and heal from trauma without specific treatment, but a substantial proportion develop persistent and sometimes disabling symptoms, including PTSD, depression, chronic physical symptoms, or substance misuse. The impact of trauma and PTSD on individuals and society is profound. In addition to distress caused by hallmark clinical symptoms, PTSD disrupts interpersonal relationships; increases the risk of depression, anxiety, and substance use disorders; increases the likelihood of high school and college failure, and teenage childbearing; and reduces the ability to work

(Davidson, 2001; Kessler, Sonnega, Bromet, Hughes, & Nelson, 1995). Moreover, PTSD frequently results in severe reductions in quality of life (Rapaport, Clary, Fayyad, & Endicott, 2005) and is associated with increased suicidality (Panagioti, Gooding, & Tarrier, 2012); those with PTSD have been shown to be 6 times more likely to attempt suicide as compared with matched controls (Kessler, Borges, & Walters, 1999). Research also indicates that physical health problems occur in excess for people with PTSD, including coronary artery disease, arthritis, asthma, and gastrointestinal symptoms (Boscarino, 1997, 2006). As a result, a high proportion of those with PTSD must simultaneously cope with other psychiatric diagnoses in addition to chronic pain or other symptoms because of medical problems. For people with PTSD, comorbidity is the norm rather than the exception.

To help individuals with PTSD, treatments have been successfully developed, studied, and refined over the past 3 decades. As a result, therapies with proven efficacy, such as cognitive processing therapy (CPT), prolonged exposure therapy (PE), and eye movement desensitization and reprocessing (EMDR), are now available to help treat symptoms of PTSD.

So, why are improved or additional strategies needed, despite significant advances in the field? They are necessary because many individuals continue to experience PTSD symptoms after taking part in evidence-based approaches (Bradley, Greene, Russ, Dutra, & Westen, 2005; Steenkamp, Litz, Hoge, & Marmar, 2015) or they have other symptoms not adequately addressed by existing treatments. As discussed in Chapter 1, the spectrum of clinical manifestations in PTSD is broad, and a one-size-fits-all approach is unlikely to meet the needs of all people (Cloitre, 2015). In addition, the range of available treatments does not necessarily match the range of preferences of people with trauma, which could affect the level of engagement in care, which in turn could influence outcomes (e.g., some people may prefer to start treatment with an approach focused on their trauma, whereas others may prefer a non-trauma-focused approach). The complexity of needs and wide spectrum of symptoms of people with PTSD has spawned efforts to develop new treatment approaches, driven by interest among both clinicians and patients. The purpose of this book is to explicate one category of additional treatment for PTSD that holds the potential to meet some of the challenges faced by individuals with PTSD—interventions based on teaching mindfulness.

In MBIs the emphasis is on changing the *relationship* to thoughts, emotions, bodily sensations, and associated behaviors. MBIs attempt to enhance the ability to attend to experience with an attitude of nonjudgment, curiosity, openness, acceptance, and kindness (Kabat-Zinn, 2009; Siegel, 2007).

By shaping how and where attention is placed, and by providing a framework for understanding the nature of thoughts, emotions, and sensations, increased mindfulness is theorized to foster more adaptive responses to stress and pain (Baer, 2003). In MBIs, group leaders or therapists do not explicitly attempt to provide techniques or guidance to change thoughts, beliefs, or behaviors. Instead, the sessions focus on bringing nonjudgmental attention to present-moment experience with an attitude of curiosity and openness. The core method of bolstering these abilities in most MBIs is through mindfulness meditation practices, such as breathing meditation, body scan meditation, or mindful movement (e.g., walking meditation, Tai Chi, yoga). The meditation practices in MBIs are framed as self-care practices, which participants are encouraged to utilize on a regular basis after finishing the course.

Examples of MBIs based on teaching mindfulness meditation include mindfulness-based stress reduction (MBSR), mindfulness-based cognitive therapy (MBCT) as well as many other meditation-based approaches adapted to specific conditions (Bowen et al., 2009; Duncan & Bardacke, 2010; Kristeller, Wolever, & Sheets, 2014). We focus on MBIs that emphasize meditation practices, although we recognize that other interventions with a strong evidence base for conditions other than PTSD, such as acceptance and commitment therapy (ACT) and dialectical behavioral therapy (DBT), teach mindfulness through techniques other than meditation (Hayes, Strosahl, & Wilson, 1999; Lynch, Chapman, Rosenthal, Kuo, & Linehan, 2006). The book is not focused on a specific MBI, such as MBSR; instead, we discuss general principles that we think are applicable to all interventions with a core focus of mindfulness meditation. Our goal is to provide the reader with a working knowledge of how mindfulness can be applied to conditions that commonly occur following trauma, including PTSD, depression, chronic pain, and substance use disorders. We provide a synopsis of the conceptual framework for MBIs for each of these conditions, review the current state of the literature, and offer practical suggestions aimed at helping clinicians to effectively offer MBIs to people with trauma.

For PTSD, the literature on MBIs is still in a nascent state, and the evidence base does not allow us to draw firm conclusions on the efficacy of MBIs for PTSD. However, there is some evidence of benefit for PTSD and other conditions that commonly occur following trauma, and to date there is little evidence to suggest harm. So, why write a book now? One reason is that, despite the need for definitive clinical trials, MBIs are increasingly offered to populations with PTSD. For example, 77% of specialty programs for PTSD in the VA now offer some type of mindfulness training (Libby,

Pilver, & Desai, 2012). Also, the application of MBIs to PTSD by clinicians has been buoyed by the recognition that—at least in theory—mindfulness practice provides gentle, gradual techniques that run counter to deeply ingrained symptoms of chronic PTSD. For example, in mindfulness practice, rather than avoiding distressing situations, a person is encouraged to notice reactivity and regard such experiences with curiosity and openness. Rather than ruminating and attempting to problem-solve difficulties, a person is encouraged to learn how to set those habits aside and "be with" perceived problems. Rather than reacting to distressing stimuli, a person is encouraged to recognize and disengage from habitual patterns. Rather than suppressing unpleasant feelings, a person is encouraged to feel what they feel—even if it is difficult to bear. And rather than being discouraged by shame and guilt, a person is encouraged to acknowledge and allow these experiences with an attitude of kindness and nonjudgment. Whether MBIs can fulfill the above potentialities remains to be seen, as we discuss in the chapters that follow.

Our clinical experience tells us that the upsurge in interest in MBIs for PTSD and trauma is in part driven by the fact that patients with PTSD are often seeking help for multiple challenges, including chronic pain, depression, and substance use disorders, on top of other life difficulties such as poverty, isolation, and fractured family relationships. If, as the evidence suggests, MBIs simultaneously provide some measure of benefit for multiple areas of difficulty (e.g., chronic pain, substance misuse, depression, and possibly PTSD), the MBI can play an important role helping a person with PTSD gain a foothold in their struggle to cope with very challenging circumstances (Holliday et al., 2014; Kearney & Simpson, 2015). In the words of one participant with PTSD who recently completed MBSR:

> I don't feel like I'm circling the gutter now, I feel like I'm getting better and that I have a life ahead of me. So I don't attribute that all to [the mindfulness teacher], it's also [my therapist] who does the triggers and coping skills CBT course that's been incredibly helpful, but I think first and foremost, it's the combination of all three.

As this quote illustrates, we view MBIs primarily as a complement to other treatments for PTSD. In our experience, many people who have already participated in established PTSD treatments choose to participate in a MBI as a way of working with persistent difficulties, such as a loss of meaning, feelings of disconnection and alienation, or persistent emotional numbing. Others may not feel ready to participate in a trauma-focused PTSD treatment and may choose to participate in an MBI as an initial step toward working with the consequences of trauma. An enhanced ability to tolerate distressing feelings and thoughts, with an attitude of openness and kindness, may in theory be of help to them in the future if they engage in therapies specifically focused on alleviating PTSD symptoms.

In our experience, some people come to class desperate to get off their medications or at least minimize the number of medications they take. Some want an alternative to medications because they are concerned about side effects or becoming addicted. Others are interested in mind–body approaches because they understand the link between their stress and pain. Many have never tried meditation before and are open to anything that can help them, whereas others may have pursued integrative medicine approaches in the past and found them beneficial. Most individuals continue to pursue other treatment modalities (e.g., medication management, psychotherapy) while taking part in mindfulness groups and see them as a complement to their other treatments. In addition, some may be looking for help with social isolation and want a group format. Some wish to learn to deal with problems more independently. Others seek insight about their suffering related to PTSD. One participant summarized the reasons for seeking out mindfulness classes:

> I think ultimately I was looking to gain some insight and peace on the suffering that I endure from PTSD. I mean, ultimately that was the goal. I've been moderately successful managing pain through meditation on my own so I hoped maybe to get a better tool to do that with. But really the primary reason for going was because PTSD . . . the feeling of remorse, kind of depression, sadness . . . *guilt*, that's the key word. *Guilt*. And just kind of a purposeless existence.

Our intention in writing this book is to provide a resource designed both to help clinicians understand the landscape of trauma more fully and to provide practical suggestions to help group leaders effectively teach mindfulness to those who have sustained trauma. In Part I we begin by providing an overview of the landscape of trauma. Each chapter in Part I is designed to provide a working knowledge of clinical conditions that commonly occur following trauma. Chapter 1 focuses on PTSD. It provides an overview of the clinical manifestations of PTSD and discusses how mindfulness is theorized to counter many of the hallmark symptoms of PTSD. A review of the extant literature on the safety of MBIs for PTSD is provided, along with an overview and discussion of outcome studies of MBIs for PTSD. Chapter 2 reviews other posttrauma sequelae: depression, chronic pain, substance use disorders, and functional somatic syndromes. An overview of the clinical manifestations of each condition is provided along with a discussion of the theoretical basis for applying MBIs. The overarching goal of Part I is to provide readers with a working knowledge of the most common clinical manifestations of trauma and an understanding of how mindfulness can be taught in an effort to benefit these symptoms.

Part II of the book focuses on practical considerations. Chapter 3 provides tips and advice on forming and managing groups, with an emphasis on how best to teach mindfulness to individuals with PTSD, chronic pain, and depression. Suggestions for managing group dynamics are provided. In Chapter 4, specific mindfulness practices are discussed, including the body scan practice, breathing meditation, yoga, and loving-kindness meditation. Suggestions are provided about how to guide each meditation practice, including commentary on tone, content, and use of language when working with populations with PTSD. Advice and suggestions are also provided for teaching individuals with chronic pain. Chapter 5 provides a synopsis of the rationale for understanding key mechanisms involved in maintenance of posttrauma sequelae by MBI teachers and therapists, and it discusses issues surrounding teacher experience and qualifications.

It is our hope that the material presented in this book will lead to a greater understanding of how mindfulness can help mitigate factors that maintain or worsen conditions commonly experienced by trauma survivors, and that this greater understanding will translate into more effective teaching and improved outcomes for patients.

PART **I** THE LANDSCAPE
OF TRAUMA

1 WHY MINDFULNESS-BASED INTERVENTIONS FOR POSTTRAUMATIC STRESS DISORDER?

When teaching mindfulness to individuals who have sustained trauma, instructors should understand the map of the territory so that, when needed, they can provide explanations of the rationale for mindfulness along with encouragement and suggestions aimed at helping people learn the material at hand. This chapter provides a brief overview of the epidemiology of trauma exposure and PTSD in the United States, reviews the symptoms PTSD comprises, and describes how PTSD is often associated with significant impairment in multiple domains of health. The multiplicity of clinical presentations associated with PTSD is described along with a brief overview of the current gold standard treatments for PTSD, which are based on cognitive behavior therapy (CBT). The reasons why some individuals may require additional or different types of interventions to address their PTSD symptoms are described, and mindfulness-based interventions (MBIs) are introduced along with discussion of how mindfulness practice can be applied to specific manifestations of PTSD. An overview of the literature base evaluating outcomes of MBIs for PTSD is provided along with a review of what is known about the safety of MBIs for individuals with

http://dx.doi.org/10.1037/0000154-002
Mindfulness-Based Interventions for Trauma and Its Consequences, by D. J. Kearney and T. L. Simpson

PTSD. We conclude the chapter with a case presentation that illustrates many of the teaching points discussed.

EPIDEMIOLOGY OF TRAUMA AND PTSD

Most adults experience significant trauma at some point in their lives, yet only a minority develop PTSD. The frequent occurrence of trauma over the lifespan was demonstrated in a large, nationally representative U.S. survey that queried participants about 19 types of trauma (Goldstein et al., 2016). More than two thirds of the respondents reported exposure to at least one potentially traumatic event, and exposure to multiple traumas was common. The most common traumas, in descending order of frequency, were sexual abuse, seeing a dead body, intimate partner violence, and experiencing a serious or life-threatening injury or illness. Other population-based studies have found similar rates of trauma exposure (Breslau et al., 1998; Creamer, Burgess, & McFarlane, 2001; Stein, Walker, Hazen, & Forde, 1997). Across studies there is a consistent finding that women are more likely than men to have experienced rape and sexual molestation, whereas men are more likely to report nonintimate partner violence and exposure to military combat.

It should be emphasized that some distress after a traumatic event is normal. Distress in the face of trauma is considered a normal reaction to abnormal events (Friedman, Resick, & Keane, 2014; Norris, Murphy, Baker, & Perilla, 2003); for most people who experience significant distress following trauma, symptoms abate within a few months. However, a substantial subset of individuals develops PTSD in the wake of trauma exposure. Recent epidemiologic data indicate the lifetime prevalence of PTSD among men and women is 4.1% and 8.9%, respectively, while past-year prevalence is 3.2% and 6.1%, respectively (Goldstein et al., 2016).

The current diagnostic criteria for PTSD in the fifth edition of the *Diagnostic and Statistical Manual of Mental Disorders* (*DSM–5*; American Psychiatric Association, 2013) include exposure to a traumatic event along with the development of the intrusions of trauma-related memories, avoidance of trauma-related cues, negative alterations in cognitions and mood, and alterations in arousal and reactivity. *DSM–5* defines *trauma* as "actual or threatened death, serious injury, or sexual violence" (American Psychiatric Association, 2013, p. 271). The intrusions symptom cluster comprises five symptoms, at least one of which needs to be present, which are characterized by memories, images, and nightmares related to a trauma and may or may not be accompanied by strong physiological responses to the memories or to actual, tangible reminders of traumas. The avoidance symptom cluster is made up of two symptoms, at least one of which must be present to meet diagnostic criteria. These symptoms involve avoidance of trauma-related thoughts and feelings and of external trauma reminders, such as places, activities, or situations. The negative alterations in cognitions and mood cluster requires the presence of at least two of seven symptoms that have to do with loss of interest and pleasure in previously enjoyed activities, social estrangement, constricted affect, and persistent negative, typically exaggerated, beliefs about oneself, others, and the world. The final cluster, alterations in arousal and reactivity, is comprised of six symptoms, at least two of which must be present for the PTSD diagnostic criteria to be met. These symptoms tap such issues as anger and irritability, self-destructive or high-risk behaviors, poor sleep and concentration, exaggerated startle reaction, and hypervigilance. Additional diagnostic criteria include that symptoms must have persisted for more than 1 month posttrauma; not be the result of medications, substance use, or other illness; and be associated with significant distress and/or functional impairment (American Psychiatric Association, 2013). In *DSM–5*, PTSD is categorized with traumatic and stressor-related disorders rather than with the anxiety disorders; a shift based, in part, on the recognition that clinical presentations following trauma are heterogeneous and may be quite complex (American Psychiatric Association, 2013; Resick & Miller, 2009). This is illustrated by a study of people with PTSD that found only a minority experienced anxiety as their primary emotion; the remainder reported sadness, disgust, or anger as their primary emotion (Power & Fyvie, 2013). The spectrum of clinical manifestations of PTSD can also include the following subtypes: anxiety, dysphoric/anhedonic, aggressive/substance-abusing, guilt/shame/other and dissociative as well as combinations of these clinical phenotypes (Friedman et al., 2014).

In addition to contending with the symptoms associated with PTSD, people with this condition often experience additional reductions in both mental and physical health. When quality of life is measured for individuals with PTSD, the degree of impairment is often severe, with the largest impact being for mental health and social functioning (Olatunji, Cisler, & Tolin, 2007; Rapaport et al., 2005). Physical health problems also occur in excess for people with PTSD, including coronary artery disease, arthritis, asthma, and gastrointestinal symptoms (Boscarino, 1997, 2006). The overall effect is that many people with PTSD often experience reduced employability, marital instability, failure to meet their educational potential, and significant impairment in day-to-day functioning (Kessler, 2000). A diagnosis of PTSD is also associated with a significantly increased risk of attempted suicide (Kessler et al., 1999; Panagioti et al., 2012).

It is common for individuals with PTSD to have active symptoms for many years. An older study from the National Comorbidity Survey suggests a median duration of PTSD symptoms of 3 years for those who receive treatment, whereas for those who do not receive treatment, symptoms continue for a median duration of 5 years (Kessler et al., 1995). However, these estimates—which demonstrate years of symptoms related to a traumatic event—do not fully describe the profound burden of PTSD over the lifespan given that many people with PTSD experience multiple traumas (Breslau et al., 1998; Karam et al., 2014). Experiencing additional traumas often leads to additional episodes of PTSD, and each episode can result in years of symptoms. A review of longitudinal studies involving clinical and community groups with PTSD found that people exposed to recurring traumas (e.g., war veterans, first responders, Holocaust survivors) were more likely to have chronic courses than those whose posttrauma circumstances changed significantly (e.g., refugee groups able to resettle in peaceful countries; Steinert, Hofmann, Leichsenring, & Kruse, 2015). When multiple traumas are considered, it is estimated that the typical person with PTSD endures active symptoms for more than 20 years during his or her lifetime (Kessler, 2000).

ESTABLISHED PSYCHOLOGICAL TREATMENTS FOR PTSD

People with PTSD seek help in a variety of ways. The National Comorbidity Survey Replication study estimated that 50% of people with PTSD received some form of treatment in the health care system within the prior 12 months, most commonly through a mental health provider (34%) or a general medical provider (31%; Wang et al., 2005). Additionally, nearly a quarter of people with PTSD report having attended self-help groups at some point in their lives to address mental health concerns other than substance use problems (Simpson, Rise, Browne, Lehavot, & Kaysen, 2019). The relatively low rate of help seeking for PTSD is likely because of multiple factors, including the stigma of mental illness, the expense of treatment, a person's belief that she or he does not have a significant problem, or the belief that the problem will get better on its own (Kessler, 2000; Wang et al., 2005). Additionally, given that PTSD is characterized by avoidance of trauma reminders, lack of trust in others, and shame and guilt, it is not surprising that many people avoid treatment. Along these same lines, the nature of PTSD may lead people to feel they are either undeserving of help or beyond help.

Fortunately, a number of psychological therapies for PTSD have been found to be helpful in reducing or alleviating distressing symptoms associated with it. Multiple treatment guidelines exist for PTSD, and they recommend several specific interventions for PTSD, including prolonged exposure (PE), cognitive processing therapy (CPT), eye movement desensitization and reprocessing (EMDR), stress-inoculation training (SIT), and present-centered therapy (PCT; Bisson, Roberts, Andrew, Cooper, & Lewis, 2013; "VA/DoD Clinical Practice Guidelines," 2017). On the basis of numerous high-quality studies that demonstrate the long-term efficacy of PE and CPT, there is general agreement across guidelines endorsing these interventions as first-line treatments for PTSD (Powers, Halpern, Ferenschak, Gillihan, & Foa, 2010; Resick, Williams, Suvak, Monson, & Gradus, 2012; "VA/DoD Clinical Practice Guidelines," 2017). PE is a form of CBT that includes elements of psychoeducation, imaginal exposure, in vivo exposure to fear-producing trauma-related stimuli and processing of trauma memories (van Minnen, Harned, Zoellner, & Mills, 2012). CPT is a CBT designed to provide skills to process maladaptive cognitions and beliefs (Resick et al., 2015; Watts et al., 2013). Both have undergone successful dissemination based on proven efficacy (Hundt, Harik, Thompson, Barrera, & Miles, 2018).

Psychological treatments for PTSD can be broadly categorized as trauma focused or non-trauma-focused. Trauma-focused therapies (e.g., PE, CPT, EMDR) help those with PTSD process trauma-related memories, thoughts, emotions, and beliefs. In contrast, non-trauma-focused therapies do not directly address trauma-related emotions, beliefs, and memories. Rather, most of these interventions (e.g., stress-inoculation training; Meichenbaum, 2007) place emphasis on acquiring skills for stress management and problem-solving in daily life (Frost, Laska, & Wampold, 2014; Meichenbaum, 2017). PCT is another non-trauma-focused therapy that helps individuals with PTSD identify the symptoms that interfere with their quality of life and functionality and then draws ideas for problem solving from the patient with an emphasis on successful past coping (Shea & Schnurr, 2017). Evidence from meta-analyses indicates that non-trauma-focused interventions, including PCT, result in clinically meaningful improvements in PTSD symptoms with medium to large effect sizes (Dorrepaal et al., 2014; Frost et al., 2014; Steenkamp et al., 2015). There is also evidence suggesting that PCT (Frost et al., 2014; Imel, Laska, Jakupcak, & Simpson, 2013) and interpersonal psychotherapy for PTSD (Markowitz et al., 2015) may have lower dropout rates than trauma-focused treatments. Additionally, a significant subset of patients does not benefit from CBT-oriented PTSD interventions or continue to have significant residual PTSD symptoms (Bradley et al., 2005; Steenkamp et al., 2015), and recognition of this has spurred the search for additional or complementary treatments.

MBIs FOR PTSD

In theory, if patients are offered treatments that match the symptoms most bothersome to them and they can do so in a way that matches their preferred starting point (e.g., beginning therapy with a technique that directly works with the trauma vs. a non-trauma-focused approach), increased engagement and improved outcomes might occur (Cloitre, 2015). Patients' interest in using complementary and alternative medicine (CAM) approaches (now preferably termed complementary and integrative health [CIH]) to help manage their PTSD appears to be increasing over time. Data from 2005 found that 13% utilized CIH, whereas a more recent survey of people with past-year PTSD found that 39% used CIH to address their emotional and mental problems, with 17.5% reporting use of meditation techniques (Kessler et al., 2005; Libby, Pilver, & Desai, 2013). For PTSD, the literature suggests that patient preferences are a key driver in increased engagement in CIH modalities for PTSD because many patients view CIH modalities as more likely to address the whole person rather than just their illness (Kroesen, Baldwin, Brooks, & Bell, 2002). Also, dissatisfaction with conventional care and reliance on prescription medications have been cited as factors motivating patients to seek out holistic, integrative perspectives (Kroesen et al., 2002) such as MBIs.

Mindfulness can be defined as "the capacity to maintain awareness of, and openness to, immediate experience—including internal mental states, thoughts, feelings, memories and impinging elements of the external world—without judgment and with acceptance" (Briere, 2015, pp. 14–15). MBIs emphasize changing a person's *relationship* to thoughts, emotions, and bodily sensations. MBIs teach meditation practices as a core method of bolstering the ability to attend to experience with an attitude of nonjudgment, patience, curiosity, trust, nonstriving, acceptance, and letting go (Kabat-Zinn, 2013). In addition to these attitudinal qualities, MBIs teach the ability to sustain, direct, and shift attention (e.g., the ability to intentionally disengage from automatic cycles of thought). MBIs also provide a framework to understand the nature of thoughts, emotions, and bodily sensations, which are presented as changing events to be regarded with acceptance and openness. Such a shift in attitudinal and attentional abilities is theorized to foster positive cognitive and behavioral change in response to stress and pain (Baer, 2003). In MBIs, group leaders or therapists do not explicitly attempt to guide participants in the process of changing thoughts, beliefs, or behaviors (beyond the behavioral change of attending class and practicing mindfulness during class and at home).

In MBIs, the primary method of enhancing the ability to attend to experience with mindful attention is through mindfulness meditation practices, such as breathing meditation, body scan meditation, eating meditation, or mindful movement (e.g., yoga, walking meditation, qi gong). The mindfulness meditation practices in MBIs are described to participants as self-care practices, which they are encouraged to continue to use long after finishing the course. Uptake of these practices appears to occur at a high rate; at least 75% report using mindfulness techniques in daily life at follow-up ranging from 6 to 48 months (Baer, 2003; Kabat-Zinn, Lipworth, Burncy, & Sellers, 1986).

MBIs have increasingly been applied in health care on the basis of supportive evidence for a variety of conditions, including chronic pain (Cherkin et al., 2016; Day, 2017; Goldberg et al., 2018; Reiner, Tibi, & Lipsitz, 2013), somatoform disorders (Lakhan & Schofield, 2013), anxiety (Hofmann, Sawyer, Witt, & Oh, 2010), addictions (Bowen et al., 2014; Brewer et al., 2009; Garland & Howard, 2018), and depression (Goldberg et al., 2018; Segal, Williams, & Teasdale, 2013). The research on MBIs in general has grown at an exponential pace, with some studies attempting to address methodological shortcomings that were common in the early literature base, although recent reviews suggest the field still has a way to go to improve the quality of MBI evaluations (Goldberg et al., 2017; Goyal et al., 2014). We include in this chapter a discussion of strengths and limitations of key studies covering the extant evidence base for MBIs for PTSD, which immediately follows an overview of the rationale for applying MBIs to PTSD.

In this book, we focus on MBIs that emphasize meditation practices, although we recognize that other interventions with a strong evidence base for conditions other than PTSD, such as acceptance and commitment therapy (ACT) and dialectical behavioral therapy (DBT), teach mindfulness through techniques other than meditation (Hayes et al., 1999; Lynch et al., 2006). Two of the most prevalent MBIs that are based on teaching mindfulness meditation are mindfulness-based stress reduction (MBSR) and mindfulness-based cognitive therapy (MBCT). In addition, many other meditation-based approaches have been adapted to the needs of specific populations. For example, among the many MBIs that have been developed are programs for substance use disorder relapse prevention, childbirth and parenting, and eating disorders (Bowen et al., 2009; Duncan & Bardacke, 2010; Kristeller et al., 2014).

THEORETICAL MODELS OF MINDFULNESS AND RELATIONSHIP TO PTSD

Several conceptual models of mindfulness have been proposed to explain MBI's effects on distress and psychiatric challenges (Hölzel et al., 2011; Shapiro, Carlson, Astin, & Freedman, 2006; Teasdale & Chaskalson, 2011a, 2011b). Although general models of mindfulness have not been evaluated specifically in the context of PTSD, these models may prove helpful in understanding how mindfulness practice leads to positive change in this setting. One model posits that mindfulness leads to benefit through a shift in perspective termed *reperceiving* (Shapiro et al., 2006), which is compatible with a number of theorized and demonstrated healthy shifts in cognition described by other investigators, including decentering (Fresco et al., 2007; Safran & Segal, 1990), metacognitive awareness (Teasdale et al., 2002), cognitive defusion (Hayes et al., 1999), and improved attention regulation (Hölzel et al., 2011).

The Shapiro model specifically posits that intention, attention, and attitude are interwoven aspects of mindfulness that lead to the metamechanism of reperceiving (i.e., a shift in perspective). In MBIs, these three interwoven aspects of mindfulness are taught in several ways. In MBIs, *intention* is often highlighted by asking participants to reflect on their motivation, or personal vision, for taking part in the MBI, along with acknowledgment that this intention can change and evolve over time. Paying *attention* is taught in MBIs through meditation practices in which a person is asked to observe his or her moment-to-moment internal or external experience. These meditation practices also seek to further develop the ability to sustain attention or shift attention. Finally, a certain *attitude* or quality of attention is emphasized in MBIs by inviting participants to pay attention without judgment and with kindness, curiosity, and openness. Together, these aspects of mindfulness foster the ability to "step back" such that patients are able to reevaluate themselves, their relations with others, and their relationship with their body, thoughts, and feelings. In Shapiro et al.'s (2006) conceptual model, reperceiving overarches the other direct mechanisms of mindfulness, which include (a) self-regulation; (b) values clarification; (c) cognitive, emotional, and behavioral flexibility; and (d) exposure.

Although this model has not been directly applied and tested in the setting of PTSD, some aspects of this framework are consistent with evidence from the trauma literature that cognitive factors (e.g., fixed posttraumatic beliefs, ruminative coping styles), as well as avoidance, serve to maintain or worsen PTSD symptomatology. For individuals who have long been burdened by symptoms characterized by reactive distress, fixed patterns of avoidance, consistently poor self-appraisal and other appraisals, and loss of meaningful engagement with others and once-valued activities, reperceiving of one's circumstance may lead to empowerment, positive changes in quality of life, and potentially to symptom reductions.

Theoretical models of mindfulness can also be described from a Buddhist perspective (Grabovac, Lau, & Willett, 2011). In the Buddhist psychological model, experience is formed by a continuous series of sense impressions and mental events, which arise rapidly and pass away. The awareness of a sense object produces a feeling tone, which can be pleasant, unpleasant, or neutral, which causes a person to pursue experiences that are pleasant (termed *attachment*) and to avoid experiences that are unpleasant (termed *aversion* or *avoidance*). Of note, in the Buddhist model, it is not the object of attention that causes attachment or aversion; attachment or aversion arises through one's responses to the feeling tone of the experience, and the feeling tone of an experience is shaped by many factors, including one's past experiences. The feelings associated with an initial sense impression produce additional mental events (i.e., thoughts and feelings), which in turn produce additional feelings; this process is termed *mental proliferation*, which fuels suffering. In the Buddhist psychological model, it is lack of awareness of reactions of attachment and aversion to pleasant, unpleasant, and neutral experiences and associated mental proliferation that maintains the process and leads to suffering (Grabovac et al., 2011).

In Buddhist theory, mindfulness involves observing the three characteristics inherent in experience: impermanence, suffering, and not-self. Such mindful observation in turn leads to insight and understanding, as well as *equanimity*, defined as a balanced state of mind in which equal interest is taken in pleasant, unpleasant, or neutral states. Insight and equanimity minimize attachment, aversion, or identification with experience and lead to reduced mental proliferation, which includes narrative or ruminative thought processes associated with experience (Grabovac et al., 2011). Concentration, enhanced attention regulation, and ethical conduct also contribute to reductions in mental proliferation. Again, this model has not been empirically tested among individuals with PTSD, but from this perspective, mindfulness may help address PTSD-related distress through reductions in avoidance of unpleasant feeling states and by reducing habitual reactions and other forms of mental proliferation (e.g., rumination, fixed posttraumatic cognitions, unhelpful narratives) that fuel suffering and increase symptomatology. The result may be not only reduced symptoms but also an expanded sense that one is neither a fixed entity nor alone and cut off from others and the world.

We turn now to an overview of how MBIs may help to address some of the chief symptoms of PTSD and common, often unhelpful, ways of coping with them.

Avoidance

Avoidance of trauma-related reminders is a major symptom of PTSD (American Psychiatric Association, 2013). Ehlers and Clark (2000) identified three types of avoidance behaviors: cognitive avoidance (trying not to think of the trauma; occupying mind at all times); emotional avoidance (controlling feelings, numbing emotions; avoiding anything that could cause positive or negative feelings); and behavioral avoidance (taking drugs, avoiding crowded places, avoiding other people; Ehlers & Clark, 2000). Avoidance behaviors also manifest in interpersonal relationships and can lead to a lack of openness and trust in others, resulting in poorer quality relationships in which misunderstanding and miscommunication are likely (Dobie et al., 2004; Gerlock, Grimesey, & Sayre, 2014; Jakupcak et al., 2011). Individuals with PTSD may also limit going places or doing things that they associate with trauma experiences to avoid feeling anxious. Although this may help to prevent distress in the short term, over time this can lead to decreased stress tolerance and an impoverished lifestyle (American Psychiatric Association, 2013).

A central focus of MBIs is cultivating an increased ability to bring mindful attention to present-moment experience, including difficult emotional states, which are prevalent in PTSD. For a trauma survivor, the ability to bring nonevaluative attention to her or his own experience, regardless of whether it is pleasant or unpleasant, as is taught in MBIs, can be considered the opposite of avoidance. An increased ability to access and directly engage psychological pain, whether through mindfulness practice or other therapies, allows distressing material to be processed, which may result in clinical improvement over time (Briere, 2015). In MBIs, participants are taught to become more aware of their patterns of reactivity, to observe these reactions without judgment, and to use mindfulness practices (e.g., breathing meditation) to manage moments of stress, anxiety, and anger. In theory, this may help them to move forward into difficult situations rather than using avoidance strategies to cope with fear or anxiety (Lang et al., 2012).

Evidence from the research literature supports reduced PTSD avoidance symptoms after participation in a MBI, particularly internal avoidance (i.e., emotional numbing; King et al., 2013; Stephenson, Simpson, Martinez, & Kearney, 2016). One study sought to clarify the question of which aspects of mindfulness practice benefit specific symptoms of PTSD by examining the association between changes in specific facets of mindfulness (defined by the Five Facet Mindfulness Questionnaire [FFMQ]) and PTSD symptom clusters over the course of treatment with an MBI (Stephenson et al., 2016). As measured by the FFMQ, mindfulness includes five facets: acting with awareness, observing, describing, nonreactivity, and nonjudgment. The change in each of these facets of the FFMQ was examined in relation to changes in PTSD symptoms (reexperiencing, avoidance, emotional numbing, hyperarousal). The results indicated that increases in acting with awareness (i.e., being aware of one's present-moment experience) and nonreactivity were the two facets of mindfulness most strongly associated with reductions in PTSD clinical symptoms, with the strongest associations for reductions in emotional numbing and hyperarousal.

Mindfulness may also function as a form of exposure that could temper the fear and avoidance that are clinical hallmarks of PTSD. Preliminary evidence for this proposition comes from findings that fear extinction is associated with mindfulness practice but not with instruction to simply relax (Kummar, 2018). When referring to MBIs as a form of exposure therapy, understand that in MBIs (in contradistinction to PE), no attempt is made to specifically reactivate trauma-related memories or content. Instead, in MBIs a person is asked to notice whatever thoughts, emotions, and body sensations arise in the present (including difficult or strong emotions) without a specific attempt to bring trauma-related material to the surface. The practice of stepping back and observing difficult thoughts, emotions, and sensations that arise in the course of mindfulness practice is theorized to gradually lead to "extinction of fear responses and avoidance behaviors previously elicited by these stimuli" (Baer, 2003, p. 129).

Hyperarousal

Hypervigilance is a core aspect of the hyperarousal PTSD symptom criterion and is defined as excessive perception of threat-related information in the environment (Dalgleish, Moradi, Taghavi, Neshat-Doost, & Yule, 2001). Individuals with PTSD tend to be hyperaware of and sensitive to potentially threatening cues, with a reduced threshold for threat, such that cues that are nonthreatening are perceived as dangerous (Dalgleish et al., 2001). Threat-related information is more likely to be processed, maintaining the disorder in a feedback loop, while nonthreatening information is less likely to be processed. Paradoxically, despite being on guard and scanning for threat, people with PTSD are prone to exaggerated startle reactions. Additionally, those with PTSD are apt to respond to others and to situational challenges with irritability and anger, and they often have difficulty concentrating and falling and staying asleep (Boyd, Lanius, & McKinnon, 2018).

Mindfulness is thought to have potential utility in addressing these issues because it teaches individuals to utilize mindfulness practices as a means of adopting a nonreactive stance to distressing aspects of experience. Such nonreactivity is hypothesized to facilitate learning that can lead to extinction of fear responses previously elicited by these stimuli (Shapiro et al., 2006). Interventional studies demonstrate that mindfulness interventions reduce physiological arousal and reactivity to stress (Vujanovic, Niles, Pietrefesa, Schmertz, & Potter, 2013). In a before-and-after study of MBSR for veterans, all PTSD symptom clusters decreased significantly over time, but hyperarousal exhibited the largest change (Kearney, McDermott, Malte, Martinez, & Simpson, 2013). Correlational studies also suggest a relationship between mindfulness and hyperarousal (Chopko & Schwartz, 2013; Wahbeh, Lu, & Oken, 2011). As described above, in a study that assessed which facets of mindfulness were associated with reductions in specific symptoms of PTSD, nonreactivity and acting with awareness were associated with reductions in hyperarousal and emotional numbing (Stephenson et al., 2016).

Posttraumatic Cognitions and Beliefs

One of the core features of PTSD involves negative changes in thoughts and mood such that following trauma many people develop negative fixed beliefs about self, others, and the world in general that can lead to added suffering. Table 1.1 provides examples of common beliefs and attitudes associated with trauma that can become entrenched in the setting of PTSD.

A fundamental capacity developed by mindfulness practice is the ability to step back from one's thoughts, emotions, and sensations and view them from a new perspective (Shapiro et al., 2006). Thus, mindfulness may help individuals to develop a decentered perspective, in which thoughts are seen as temporary events in the mind and not as reflections of self (Fresco et al., 2007; Safran & Segal, 1990). Regarding thoughts with curiosity and openness holds the potential to reduce distress from and reactivity to thoughts and beliefs that develop after trauma.

TABLE 1.1. Common Beliefs and Attitudes Following a Traumatic Event

Circumstance	Beliefs and attitudes
Fact that the trauma happened to me	"Nowhere is safe." "I deserved it. I don't deserve to be happy." "I can't trust anyone." "People who appear to be generous have other motives."
Initial posttraumatic stress disorder symptoms that often persist (e.g., irritability, emotional numbing, flashbacks, difficulty concentrating)	"I'm dead inside." "No one will ever understand me." "I cannot cope with stress."
Other people's reactions after trauma	"They think I am too weak to cope." "I need to appear strong." "They think what happened was my fault." "They just want me to get over it."
Other consequences of trauma (physical, social)	"My body is ruined." "I will never be able to lead a normal life again." "I am unable to feel close to anyone." "I cannot love others again." "I'm unlovable." "I'm damaged, broken."

Note. From "A Cognitive Model of Posttraumatic Stress Disorder," by A. Ehlers and D. M. Clark, 2000, *Behaviour Research and Therapy, 38*, p. 322. Copyright 2000 by Elsevier. Adapted with permission.

Pervasive feelings of shame and guilt, which often arise in the context of negative posttraumatic cognitions and beliefs, are common among people with PTSD and are theorized to play a key role in the development and maintenance of the disorder (D. A. Lee, Scragg, & Turner, 2001). Shame and guilt can be very limiting because they often affect social identify, attenuate help-seeking, and interfere with emotional processing of traumatic events (D. A. Lee et al., 2001). Feelings of shame can be a focus of rumination (Gilbert & Procter, 2006) and may also lead to a feeling of current threat through an attack on personal integrity (D. A. Lee et al., 2001). Shame can also include feelings of powerlessness, inferiority, unattractiveness, and a desire to hide perceived deficiencies (Gilbert & Procter, 2006). Guilt can occur when a person acted or failed to act in ways that they believe conflicts with their code of conduct (D. A. Lee et al., 2001), which is not an uncommon occurrence during trauma situations (Norman et al., 2018).

Mindfulness practice is hypothesized to re-create or create a safe holding environment (Epstein, 2013) in which difficult emotional experiences (e.g., shame, guilt) can be regarded with acceptance, kindness, and self-compassion, which may prove particularly helpful when kindness and support are lacking in the environment. There is preliminary evidence that mindfulness practice reduces shame in trauma survivors (Goldsmith et al., 2014). Through mindfulness practice, an increased ability to self-modulate pervasive feelings of shame, guilt, and inferiority may help to restore or establish a sense of connection to the sense of self that has been lost through traumatic experiences or that never developed if trauma happened early in life. This increased comfort with oneself may in turn, allow for reconnection (or connection) with the community as well.

Rumination is a common cognitively based response to trauma, particularly among those with more severe PTSD symptoms (Bennett & Wells, 2010; Ehring, Szeimies, & Schaffrick, 2009). Rumination can be conceived of as a specific way of relating to mental content (Ramel, Goldin, Carmona, & McQuaid, 2004) characterized by a passive and repetitive focus on negative thoughts and emotions. For individuals with PTSD, frequent revisiting of trauma memories, posttraumatic cognitions, beliefs, and feelings can add to distress and the perception of being painfully stuck. Rumination is a key factor in relapse of depression, and for this reason we cover it in additional detail in Chapter 2, this volume. For people with PTSD, there is evidence that rumination is associated with more severe PTSD symptoms (Bennett & Wells, 2010; Ehring et al., 2009; Viana et al., 2017). Although not tested in a population with PTSD, there is some experimental evidence (Williams, 2008) as well as preliminary clinical findings (Chesin et al., 2016) that mindfulness training reduces rumination in other clinical samples. The significance of rumination has also been highlighted by theorists who posit that PTSD may be more accurately characterized by anhedonic mood and anxious rumination than by pathologic fear and externalizing (Resick & Miller, 2009).

In mindfulness practice, when memories of painful past events arise, a person is encouraged to bring mindful attention to the experience, which acknowledges the reality that painful events happened, but without the repetitive patterns of thought that worsen distress. Such cognitive shifts could, in theory, enhance the ability to tolerate the discomfort of reevaluating painful past experiences and lead to changes in perspective toward those experiences, themselves, and others. Learning to disengage from cycles of rumination involves what Kabat-Zinn (2013) described as "letting go" (p. 40), wherein mindfulness practitioners are encouraged to allow experience to be as it is through the process of observing experience from moment to moment. Mindfulness practitioners learn to recognize elaborative, ruminative tendencies and repeatedly let go, or disengage, then return to the object of meditation (e.g., the breath). Through this process, participants are taught to step out of entrenched patterns of ruminative thinking.

MBIs AND PTSD: A REVIEW OF THE EVIDENCE

Three papers published since 2016 provide systematic reviews of the extant randomized clinical trials (RCTs) evaluating MBI interventions for those with current PTSD (Gallegos, Crean, Pigeon, & Heffner, 2017; Hilton et al., 2016; Niles et al., 2018), two of which also include meta-analyses (Gallegos et al., 2017; Hilton et al., 2016). All three papers included a variety of MBI approaches ranging from mantram repetition practices (i.e., to include transcendental meditation [TM]), to yoga, to MBSR. Hilton et al. (Hilton et al., 2016) combined results from eight trials representing a variety of MBI approaches and found an overall standardized mean difference (*SMD*), which is a measure of effect size and equivalent to Cohen's *d*, of -0.41 (95% CI [-0.81, -0.01]) indicating a small to medium effect on PTSD symptomatology in favor of MBIs relative to comparison conditions. The authors found that the three MBI types (i.e., mantram repetition, yoga, MBSR) did not differ significantly from one another regarding relative efficacy.

The Gallegos et al. (2017) meta-analysis separated the mindfulness MBIs, which were based primarily on MBSR, from both the yoga and the other meditation-based MBIs, which were based primarily on mantram repetition (Gallegos et al., 2017). Across the nine mindfulness MBI RCTs for PTSD that were included, the effect size was -0.34 ($p < .001$, 95% CI [-0.49, -0.18]), again indicating a small to medium effect for mindfulness MBIs. To contextualize the results of their meta-analysis, Gallegos et al. (2017) provided information from a prominent meta-analysis (Bisson et al., 2013) on the effect sizes associated with individually delivered trauma-focused and nontrauma CBT interventions for PTSD, both of which were large (Cohen's *d*s of -1.62 and -1.22, respectively). The authors also noted that the effect size associated with MBIs is comparable with that found for medication management, which is recommended as a second-line treatment for PTSD (U.S. Department of Veterans Affairs, 2017). They concluded that all three types of MBIs likely provide some benefit, increase patient choice, and because they are typically group based, may be a cost-effective complement to CBT interventions for PTSD.

The systematic reviews accompanying both meta-analyses as well as the Niles et al. (2018) systematic review echo the findings from the meta-analyses. Further, all three papers caution that there is marked heterogeneity across studies in terms of outcomes and that, overall, the quality of the extant RCTs evaluating MBIs is weak. Methodological problems that were highlighted include generally small sample sizes, failure to use intent-to-treat analytic models, short follow-up assessment windows, lack of active comparators, and failure to state an a priori power calculation (see Hilton et al., 2016, for details regarding study quality). Niles et al. (2018) specifically cautioned that because many of the extant MBI studies for those with PTSD involved small samples, there is concern that negative trials may not be published, resulting in the "file drawer effect." This concern is amplified by the fact that all three reviews appear to have used standard search strategies that likely would not have yielded "gray literature" (e.g., unpublished dissertations, conference presentations, funded grants that did not result in publications), though Gallegos et al. did include results from a study that was not published at the time that has since been published (L. L. Davis et al., 2018).

Commentary on Key Trials of MBSR for PTSD

Two RCTs that evaluated MBSR for PTSD (L. L. Davis et al., 2018; Polusny et al., 2015) merit particular attention; both are relatively large, and both compared MBSR with an active intervention, PCT, which as noted earlier is considered an empirically supported alternative for treating PTSD. The use of PCT as an active, credible comparator is an important design strength of both studies because it at least partly controls for changes that may be due to positive expectancy, relationship with the group leader, and other nonspecific elements (Palpacuer et al., 2017; Wampold & Imel, 2015). Key features of both studies, including findings and methodological strengths and weaknesses, may be found in Table 1.2.

The Polusny et al. (2015) study randomized 116 combat veterans to receive group-based standard format MBSR or standard format PCT. Although the first MBSR session included supplemental education about PTSD and an explanation of the treatment rationale, the remainder of the course was delivered without modification of the meditation practices, which included the standard duration for body scan meditation, sitting meditation, and mindful yoga. An experienced MBSR instructor led the MBSR groups, and daily homework was assigned in the form of guided meditations. Experienced group leaders led the PCT groups. Fidelity of both interventions was

TABLE 1.2. Key Features of L. L. Davis et al. (2018) and Polusny et al. (2015) Studies

Study	Participants	MBSR	PCT	Assessments	Outcomes	Safety
L. L. Davis et al., 2018	214 veterans with PTSD 191 included in analyses (attended at least one session)	1.5 hours weekly for 8 weeks plus 6-hour retreat	1.5 hours weekly for 8 weeks plus lunch gathering	Posttreatment 2-month	PTSD symptom severity Depression, mindfulness, attendance	MBSR: 5 unrelated serious adverse events PCT: 2 unrelated serious adverse events

Findings

PTSD Outcomes: The groups were not found to differ on PTSD severity as measured by the CAPS (primary outcome) at either time point, but PCL results showed a significant difference favoring MBSR at immediate posttest. Both groups saw clinically significant responses (i.e, ↓30% point drop on CAPS; MBSR: 45.2%; PCT: 37.7%, *ns*) and remission rates (i.e., } 45 on CAPS; MBSR: 30.7%; PCT: 27.3%, *ns*).

Depression: No between-groups differences on the PHQ-9, and little change from baseline to posttreatment or 2-month follow-up.

Mindfulness: No between-groups differences on Five-Factor Mindfulness Questionnaire scores; both reported small increase in mindfulness from baseline to 2-month follow-up.

Attendance: No between-groups differences on overall number of sessions attended, but 31.2% of MBSR participants completed 7&sessions vs. 58.9% of PCT participants (the difference was not tested by the authors).

Strengths and Limitations

Strengths: Large sample size; comparability of time/attention across conditions; fidelity of treatment delivery evaluated; Type I error control for secondary analyses; assessors blind to treatment assignment; use of gold standard PTSD assessment; randomization done electronically; groups were comparable at baseline; provided a priori power analysis; provided information on safety.

Limitations: Modified intent-to-treat analyses that may be sensitive to treatment assignment; alteration of standard MBSR; short follow-up duration.

(table continues)

TABLE 1.2. (continued).

Study	Participants	MBSR	PCT	Assessments	Outcomes	Safety
Polusny et al., 2015	116 veterans with PTSD	2.5 hours weekly for 8 weeks plus 6.5-hour retreat	9 weekly 1.5-hour sessions	Posttreatment 2-month	PTSD symptom severity Depression, quality of life, mindfulness, attendance	1 PCT participant attempted suicide

Findings

PTSD Outcomes: Both groups improved on PTSD severity as measured by the PCL (primary outcome) from baseline to 2-month follow-up; the MBSR group showed significantly greater improvement than the PCT group over time. The same pattern of results was found on the CAPS (secondary outcome). The groups did not differ on loss of diagnosis at either time point (immediate posttest: MBSR 42.3%; PCT: 43.9%; 2-month follow-up: MBSR: 53.3%; PCT 47.3%). Significantly more participants in MBSR had a clinically meaningful decrease in PCL score (10+ reduction) at 2-month follow-up than those in PCT (48.9% vs. 28.1%, respectively).

Depression: No between-groups differences on the PHQ-9, and little change from baseline to posttreatment or 2-month follow-up.

Quality of Life: MBSR participants reported significantly greater improvements on the WHO Quality of Life-Brief measure than PCT participants at 2-month follow-up.

Mindfulness: MBSR participants reported significantly greater improvement on the Five-Factor Mindfulness Questionnaire than the PCT participants at 2-month follow-up.

Attendance: Treatment completion (attending 7+ sessions) was significantly lower in the MBSR group (77.6%) than the PCT group (93.1%).

Strengths and Limitations

Strengths: Large sample size; standard format for both interventions; fidelity of treatment delivery evaluated; intent-to-treat analyses; assessors blind to treatment assignment; randomization done electronically; a priori power calculations included.

Limitations: Interventions differed markedly on time and attention; randomization failed to yield comparable groups; short follow-up duration; Type I error was not controlled.

Note. PTSD = posttraumatic stress disorder; MBSR = mindfulness-based stress reduction; PCT = patient-centered therapy; PCL = PTSD Checklist; CAPS = Clinician-Administered PTSD Scale; PHQ-9 = 9-item Patient Health Questionnaire; WHO = World Health Organization. Data from L. L. Davis et al. (2018) and Polusny et al. (2015).

assessed over the course of the study and found to be satisfactory. Of note, although the study included PCT as an active comparator, the total length of time spent in sessions was twice as long for MBSR, raising concern that the increased provider contact in the MBSR arm may have influenced outcomes (see the critique by D. J. Lee & Hoge, 2017, and the reply by the original authors, Erbes, Thuras, Lim, & Polusny, 2017).

The results showed that though there were no significant between-groups differences at immediate posttest, those randomized to MBSR had greater improvement in PTSD symptoms on both the self-report PTSD Checklist (Weathers, Litz, Herman, Huska, & Keane, 1993) and the gold standard Clinician-Administered PTSD Scale (CAPS; Weathers, Keane, & Davidson, 2001). Additionally, significantly more of those participating in MBSR (49%) had improvement in symptoms in the range considered clinically meaningful as compared to PCT (28%) at 2 months, though there was no difference in the likelihood of losing one's PTSD diagnosis. There were no between group differences on depression at either time point, but the MBSR group reported improvements in both quality of life and mindfulness that were significantly stronger than the PCT group at the 2-month assessment. Both interventions were well tolerated with low treatment attrition rates, though those assigned to MBSR were significantly less likely to complete seven or more sessions than those in the PCT group (77.6% vs. 93.1%, respectively), and one participant in the PCT group attempted suicide (which was determined not to be related to involvement in the study).

L. L. Davis et al. (2018) randomized 214 veterans to either group-based MBSR or PCT, and the 191 who attended at least one treatment session were included in the analyses (modified intent-to-treat analyses). In light of concerns about differential time and attention across conditions, L. L. Davis et al. modified MBSR to be eight weekly 1.5-hour sessions (with a 6-hour weekend retreat) and added a lunch gathering to the eight 1.5-hour weekly PCT sessions to partially account for the MBSR retreat time. Both the MBSR and PCT groups showed clinically significant improvement at 2 months (i.e., ≥ 30% point drop on CAPS; MBSR: 45.2%; PCT: 37.7%) as well as moderately strong remission rates (i.e., } 45 on CAPS; MBSR: 30.7%; PCT: 27.3%), but there were no between-groups differences on PTSD severity as measured by the CAPS at either immediate posttest or the longer follow-up. The MBSR group did show greater improvement than the PCT group at immediate posttest on the self-report PCL. There were no between-groups differences on depression or mindfulness and neither index showed much within subject change over time. The authors did not find that the two groups differed on the number of treatment sessions attended, but calculations done with detailed information provided on session attendance suggest that the rate of treatment completion (using the same 7+ session indicator as Polusny et al., 2015) was greater for those assigned to PCT (58.9%) than for those assigned to MBSR (31.2%).

The findings from both studies suggest that MBSR, whether delivered in its standard format or an abbreviated one, yields improvement in PTSD that is at least as strong as that associated with PCT (an empirically supported treatment for PTSD). Neither study, however, tested a noninferiority hypothesis, so we do not yet know whether there are or are not meaningful differences between these two interventions. Considering both studies' important methodological strengths, the findings suggest that MBSR may be a useful alternative or complementary intervention for PTSD. With regard to these studies' strengths, both studies are far larger than the other published RCTs testing MBSR, though the Polusny et al. (2015) study was somewhat underpowered based on their a priori power calculations. Additionally, both included a valid clinician-rated assessment of PTSD, assessors were blind to study condition, and treatment fidelity was systematically evaluated and found to be good. The two studies do, however, share a critical design limitation in that the longest follow-up assessment was 2 months posttreatment, limiting our ability to gauge endurance of treatment gains over a longer time period, whether one or the other treatment does a better job of maintaining gains, and whether there might be "snowball effects" associated with either treatment such that with more time, people exposed to MBSR and/or PCT may improve even more.

It is also noteworthy that the two studies opted to handle the issue of disparate treatment time differently. The earlier Polusny et al. (2015) study delivered MBSR in its standard format (26 hours total) and PCT in its standard format (12 hours), thereby approximating how each are typically delivered in practice but sacrificing the ability to determine whether any advantage of MBSR might have been due to the greater exposure to the teacher and fellow group members. L. L. Davis et al. (2018) addressed the time and attention issue by truncating MBSR sessions to 1.5 hours and adding a nonstandard lunch gathering to the PCT intervention. Thus, while greater methodological control was asserted, it is not possible to know whether the general lack of between-groups differences found in this study was perhaps because of having curtailed the in-session meditation practice time provided in standard MBSR courses. Both studies recruited military veterans exclusively, and there are currently no well-powered RCTs evaluating MBSR for PTSD among civilians.

Other, smaller scale studies that have evaluated abbreviated versions of MBSR have found comparably modest between-groups differences. For example, Niles et al. (2012) compared an 8-week MBI (two sessions in person followed by six telehealth sessions, based on MBSR) with similar length psychoeducation sessions for PTSD among combat veterans. Although they found greater reductions in PTSD symptoms for MBI than for psychoeducation at immediate posttest, improvement in PTSD symptoms in the MBI arm waned at follow-up. Another trial randomly assigned veterans with PTSD to four 1.5-hour mindfulness training sessions adapted from MBSR that were delivered in primary care or to usual care (Possemato et al., 2016). No differences between brief mindfulness training and usual care were found, but for those who completed the experimental intervention there were significantly larger decreases in PTSD severity and depression (Possemato et al., 2016).

Evaluation of Other MBIs for PTSD

MBCT is an 8-week MBI originally derived from MBSR for prevention of depressive relapse (Segal et al., 2013), and there is preliminary information on an adapted version for PTSD. In a nonrandomized trial comparing PTSD symptom reduction following MBCT to outcomes following other non-trauma-focused groups for combat veterans with chronic PTSD ($N = 37$), MBCT participants had greater reductions in PTSD symptom scores (King et al., 2013). The greatest reductions in symptoms were seen for avoidance/numbing symptoms, and reductions in posttraumatic cognitions were also observed.

The studies previously described report on outcomes of interventions based on teaching mindfulness without a specific focus on trauma-related exposure. Given the robust evidence base for PE (Jeffreys et al., 2014; Kehle-Forbes, Meis, Spoont, & Polusny, 2016; Tuerk et al., 2011), King et al. (2016) developed an intervention that combines elements of trauma-focused exposure therapy with mindfulness training. The clinical rationale for the combined intervention, called *mindfulness-based exposure therapy* (MBET), is to teach patients mindfulness as a method of improving emotional regulation and stress tolerance, which in turn is predicted to help them engage in trauma-focused exposure therapy (King et al., 2016). MBET consists of 16 weekly 2-hour sessions that include daily mindfulness training based on MBCT, in vivo exposure from PE, PTSD psychoeducation, and self-compassion exercises. Preliminary findings from 23 combat veterans show reduced PTSD symptoms in both MBET and PCT, which were not significantly different. However, the investigators report on before-and-after functional MRI (fMRI) neuroimaging data regarding resting-state functional connectivity in the default mode network (DMN) and salience network (SN). Patients treated with MBET were found to have significantly increased DMN resting-state functional connectivity with brain regions associated with executive control; this change was not observed in the active control group (King et al., 2016). The change in functional connectivity is consistent with an increased ability to shift attention from one type of self-referential state (e.g., rumination) to another, such as experiencing sensation and interoception (e.g., attention to the breath; King et al., 2016). Overall, the study provides a possible mechanism for the beneficial impact of mindfulness interventions on emotional regulation.

COMMENTARY ON THE SAFETY OF MBIS FOR PTSD

On the basis of available evidence from clinical trials, MBIs for PTSD appear safe and generally well tolerated. Several clinical trials of MBIs for PTSD have reported no serious adverse effects of MBIs related to the MBI (Bremner et al., 2017; Cole et al., 2015; L. L. Davis et al., 2018; Goldsmith et al., 2014; Kearney, McDermott, Malte, Martinez, & Simpson, 2012, 2013; Kimbrough, Magyari, Langenberg, Chesney, & Berman, 2010; Niles et al., 2012; Polusny et al., 2015; Possemato et al., 2016). Given that PTSD symptoms fluctuate over time in the absence of specific interventions, it can be expected that individual patients in clinical trials will sometimes experience worsening of symptoms. For example, in an RCT comparing MBSR with treatment as usual ($N = 47$), Kearney et al. (2013) found that one patient in each arm of the study had an inpatient psychiatric admission related to worsening PTSD symptoms during the study period, and in a larger RCT ($N = 116$) comparing MBSR with PCT, there was one serious adverse event, as noted above (a suicide attempt), which occurred in the PCT arm (Polusny et al., 2015). In the larger L. L. Davis et al. (2018) study ($N = 214$), which also compared MBSR with PCT, among patients who attended at least one session, there were three participants randomized to MBSR hospitalized with suicidal ideation, whereas in the PCT arm one was hospitalized for suicidal ideation; all adverse events were deemed unrelated to the study procedures (L. L. Davis et al., 2018). The extant literature does not suggest that PTSD symptom exacerbation occurs as a person progresses through a mindfulness class series. For example, the Polusny et al. (2015) and L. L. Davis et al. RCTs, which measured PTSD symptoms at Weeks 3 and 6 after beginning an 8-week MBSR series, did not show a rise in average PTSD symptom score during the course of treatment.

Another piece of evidence suggesting that participation in an MBI is not problematic for individuals with severe PTSD symptoms is a study that assessed the impact of baseline PTSD severity on clinical outcomes after MBSR, which found that those with the most severe baseline PTSD had greater improvement in PTSD symptoms compared with those with less severe PTSD (Felleman, Stewart, Simpson, Heppner, & Kearney, 2016). The perceived clinical safety and benefit of MBIs for individuals with PTSD is also indicated by the widespread use of MBIs for PTSD treatment in the Department of Veterans Affairs; Libby et al. (2012) found that some type of mindfulness training is offered by 77% of specialty programs for PTSD.

Qualitative research can be useful as an additional method to assess safety and to learn of potentially unmeasured side effects from the perspective of the participant. In a qualitative study of barriers and facilitators to participation in MBSR in a veteran population with a high prevalence of trauma, PTSD symptoms were not described as a barrier to practicing mindfulness, although some individuals had an aversion to participation in groups (Martinez et al., 2015). In a subsequent qualitative analysis of 15 veterans with PTSD who participated in MBSR, no participants described exacerbation of PTSD related to mindfulness practice or reported that the practices were too difficult because of PTSD (Schure, Simpson, Martinez, Sayre, & Kearney, 2018). Themes identified by veterans with PTSD who participated in MBSR included dealing with the past, staying in the present, acceptance of adversity, breathing through stress, relaxation, and openness to self and others (Schure et al., 2018). Two additional studies that employed qualitative research methods, each involving nine individuals with PTSD who participated in MBSR, reported satisfaction with the intervention, although some participants found it difficult (Cole et al., 2015; Müller-Engelmann, Wünsch, Volk, & Steil, 2017).

The comments here are not to suggest that individual participants may not sometimes experience anxiety or distress while practicing meditation; there have been occasional reports of anxiety or distress during meditation practices for people with a history of trauma in the literature. For example, King et al. (2013) reported that two of 20 people undergoing MBCT experienced anxiety during mindfulness exercises that contributed to dropout, with an overall dropout rate of 25%, which is similar to or lower than dropout rates for other interventions for PTSD. Other anecdotal cases of distress, anxiety, and possible clinical deterioration associated with meditation have been published (Treleaven, 2018; Van Dam et al., 2018). However, anecdotal reports cannot be used to draw conclusions about the frequency of side effects, which must be determined through prospective monitoring in clinical trials or other large-scale monitoring procedures.

When a person experiences distress or troubling emotional content during a mindfulness exercise in a therapeutic milieu, it is important to remember that it does not necessarily represent an adverse event. In the treatment of PTSD, activation of trauma-related memories or fear is considered beneficial because it leads to habituation and symptom reduction over time (Foa & Kozak, 1986). When individuals with trauma experience distressing memories, emotions, images, and thoughts, participation in the mindfulness class is framed as a valuable opportunity to learn new ways of working with these experiences. Individuals with PTSD most likely experience similar forms of distress outside of the class setting, and working with unpleasant memories, thoughts, and emotions in class, aided by a skilled mindfulness instructor and supportive group, can be considered an opportunity to learn new habits of responding. We suggest providing meditation instructions that include wording that seeks a balance between wise effort and safety; participants are encouraged to trust their intrinsic wisdom and sometimes pause, stop meditation practice, or pull back in their effort if it feels wise, and to do so without judgment. These considerations are discussed in more detail in Chapter 4. Overall, our impression, based on the extant clinical literature described in this chapter and clinical experience, is that the level of trauma-related distress experienced in MBIs is clinically acceptable and does not lead to excessive dropout, symptom exacerbation, or suicidality.

In our experience, based on thousands of clinical encounters teaching MBSR to veterans with PTSD over an approximately 10-year period, in the rare instances when a person reported trauma-related memories or distress associated with the mindfulness practices, it was possible to suggest subtle modifications or alternate practices, which allowed the person to continue and successfully complete the course. We have not had veterans with PTSD report flashbacks or other forms of dissociation during MBSR practices, which is consistent with reports of safety in clinical trials reported above. In clinical practice, we routinely frame the discussion of whether to participate in an intervention in terms of the potential risk versus the potential benefit for an individual patient. In the case of PTSD, harm has not been shown in prospective clinical trials as a result of participating in an MBI, and there is some evidence of modest benefit, as reported in the meta-analyses above. Our overall impression is that the practices are generally well tolerated by individuals with trauma, and that people with PTSD are often strongly motivated to practice mindfulness meditation despite finding the process to be difficult at times.

SUMMARY

Trauma exposure is the norm, and although most people do not go on to develop PTSD, a substantial proportion do, and their symptoms may become chronic, particularly in the face of additional trauma exposures. There are several empirically supported CBT-based interventions available to treat PTSD, and the extant literature suggests that MBIs may serve as alternatives or complements to these treatments in that they are safe, well-tolerated, and appear to result in as much symptom reduction as PCT, a non-trauma-focused CBT intervention. However, more rigorous trial designs (e.g., noninferiority trials) with larger samples and longer follow-up are needed. In addition, thoughtful consideration of treatment time/attention issues and inclusion of more varied study samples are necessary to evaluate the true promise of MBIs for treating PTSD.

In Chapter 2, we provide an overview of other common sequelae associated with trauma exposure–depression, chronic pain syndromes, and substance use disorders–and discuss the rationale for applying MBIs in these clinical settings. The extant MBI treatment outcome base for each type of condition is also summarized, along with the strengths and limitations of these literatures.

2

MINDFULNESS-BASED INTERVENTIONS FOR SELECTED CONSEQUENCES OF TRAUMA

Many people with trauma and posttraumatic stress disorder (PTSD) who attend mindfulness courses are contending with a variety of additional challenges, including other mental health and medical problems, as well as the life stress of attempting to deal with multiple conditions. Some are dealing with chronic pain and conditions such as fibromyalgia and irritable bowel syndrome (IBS), or are simultaneously trying to cope with depression or substance misuse. In the previous chapter, we gave an overview of PTSD, discussed how mindfulness practice in theory holds the potential to reduce cardinal symptoms of PTSD, and reviewed the literature on outcome studies of MBIs for PTSD. In this chapter, we provide an overview of the mindfulness-based treatment literature as it pertains to psychiatric and physical conditions that commonly co-occur with PTSD.

This chapter is included because patients do not segregate themselves cleanly by individual diagnoses. When we work with people who have sustained trauma, the norm is for them to present with multiple conditions simultaneously, and the ideal intervention would afford benefit across conditions. In the sections that follow, we review the theoretical framework

http://dx.doi.org/10.1037/0000154-003
Mindfulness-Based Interventions for Trauma and Its Consequences, by D. J. Kearney and T. L. Simpson

and evidence base for applying mindfulness practice to depression, substance misuse, chronic pain, and other functional somatic syndromes, each of which commonly occurs in conjunction with PTSD. Our aim is to provide readers a working knowledge of how mindfulness is understood to benefit individuals with each condition, with an overarching goal of helping group leaders to better teach mindfulness to people with these conditions. This chapter is intended to convey a working knowledge of the principles and putative mechanisms of change before we move on to practical issues and suggestions for effective teaching, which are described in Part II of the book (Chapters 3 and 4).

OVERVIEW OF COMORBIDITY FOLLOWING TRAUMA

The research literature confirms that people with PTSD are more likely than not to struggle with both mental and physical health issues, and many of them are likely to seek out either traditional interventions (e.g., psychotherapies and medications), complementary and integrative (CIH) modalities, or both. A large-scale epidemiological study involving over 36,000 people ages 18 years and older in the United States found that those with lifetime PTSD diagnoses were at elevated risk of a host of concomitant psychiatric conditions relative to those without PTSD (Goldstein et al., 2016). Specifically, compared with people without PTSD, those with the disorder were 3 times more likely to have a mood disorder, over 2.5 times more likely to have an anxiety disorder, 1.5 times more likely to have a substance use disorder, and nearly 3 times more likely to meet criteria for borderline personality disorder. Those with PTSD also reported markedly poorer social functioning than those without PTSD.

Similarly, a high proportion of those with PTSD deal with chronic pain and other chronic medical problems. A meta-analysis of 71 studies examined the association of trauma with somatic syndromes, including fibromyalgia, chronic widespread pain, chronic fatigue, temporomandibular joint dysfunction, and IBS and found that PTSD had a strong association with these diagnoses (Afari et al., 2014). An extensive review of the relationship between chronic pain and anxiety disorders, including PTSD (Asmundson & Katz, 2009), found that between 30% and 80% of people seeking treatment for PTSD report chronic pain. This same review estimated that those with PTSD are 2.5 times more likely than those without PTSD to have a chronic pain condition and approximately twice as likely to have other somatic conditions, including gastrointestinal conditions such as IBS.

Considering the challenges often faced by trauma survivors who participate in MBI classes, we find it critical to remember that the individuals in the room are strong and resilient. As an example, one of our past students was a paraplegic who was in constant pain but nevertheless attended every class. During the movement exercises, he spent his time in sitting meditation. Even with his significant physical limitation, he found that the class helped him immensely, and the other members of the group were moved and inspired by his tenacity. Another person had severe neuropathy, which he described as a feeling of "constantly walking on glass." He completed the program and reported that it helped him to learn new ways of coping with pain. Thus, we have found that regardless of the level of physical ability, people can take part in a mindfulness program. We have also found that people who come to mindfulness classes with very heavy mental health burdens, including significant symptoms of depression and substance misuse in addition to PTSD, are able to successfully participate in MBIs.

DEPRESSION

Individuals with PTSD are at greatly elevated risk of having concomitant depression such that they are approximately 60% more likely to meet criteria for a major depressive disorder than people without PTSD (Goldstein et al., 2016). Hence, when joining a mindfulness group, people with PTSD often are not only seeking help with PTSD but also searching for relief from their depression. Major depression is characterized by depressed mood and/or reduced interest and enjoyment in activities, sleep disturbances, fatigue, feelings of worthlessness, psychomotor agitation or retardation, reduced concentration, and suicidal ideation (American Psychiatric Association, 2013). At least five symptoms must be present during the same 2-week period, and at least one of the symptoms must be depressed mood or diminished interest/enjoyment in activities. Not only is depression painful in and of itself, it is often associated with disability, reduced functioning, lower quality of life, higher risk of co-occurring pain, anxiety, and substance-use disorders (Kamenov, Mellor-Marsá, Leal, Ayuso-Mateos, & Cabello, 2014). Thus, the burden of depression goes far beyond depressed mood and importantly, also places people at elevated risk of suicide (Chesney, Goodwin, & Fazel, 2014). Major depression also has a very high recurrence rate, with rates of recurrence of 50% after the first episode, 70% after the second, and 90% after the third (U.S. Department of Veterans Affairs, 2016). Currently, long-term maintenance antidepressants are the mainstay of treatment for prevention of relapse (U.S. Department of Veterans Affairs, 2016). However, many people report dissatisfaction with medications and prefer nonpharmacologic treatments, including holistic, integrative approaches (Kroesen et al., 2002), which has led to the study of MBIs as a strategy both for treatment of current depression and prevention of relapse.

Mindfulness and Pathways of Change for Depression

In this section, we review the rationale and impressive body of evidence indicating that mindfulness significantly reshapes the clinical course of depression. Depression is discussed in detail, given that it is a common posttrauma sequela and the mechanisms of change are more completely understood than for other applications of MBIs. Fundamentally, the mechanisms described all point to a change in the relationship to thoughts that occurs with mindfulness practice. We examine each mechanism in detail, beginning with changes in rumination. In clinical practice, our experience is that understanding the mechanisms described here is helpful when working not only with people with major depressive disorder but also with people across a broad range of symptomatology.

Rumination

Rumination is a key factor in the initial onset of depression in healthy people without a prior history of depression and similarly plays an important role in relapse and maintenance of major depression (Deyo, Wilson, Ong, & Koopman, 2009; Nolen-Hoeksema, 2000). It also predicts symptoms of anxiety (Nolen-Hoeksema, 2000) and is associated with more severe PTSD symptoms (Bennett & Wells, 2010; Ehring et al., 2009; Viana et al., 2017). As was briefly introduced in Chapter 1, rumination pertains to how one relates to mental content (Ramel et al., 2004) in ways that are passive and repetitive. There are often thoughts about the meanings of symptoms or distress, as well as thoughts about how to change one's situation (Deyo et al., 2009; Nolen-Hoeksema, 2000). For some people, rumination is a consistent style of response to depressed mood, which confers a vulnerability to depression, making it more likely that mild, transient episodes of low mood will progress to prolonged and severe episodes of depression. Rumination can remain dormant during periods without depression, but when low mood occurs, a ruminative mode of mind engages automatically. The tendency to reactivate a ruminative coping style is most pronounced among individuals with multiple episodes of depression (Segal et al., 2013).

Rumination can appear to be a logical approach to rid oneself of low mood, and the motivation to continue rumination can be strong given that it is engaged in service of the important personal goal of ending a period of unhappiness. Unfortunately, rumination usually has the counterproductive effect of perpetuating the very mood it is attempting to ameliorate. As a person ruminates over depressed mood, further lowering of mood often occurs, which in turn generates more depressive style of thinking and additional lowering of mood (Nolen-Hoeksema, 1991; Segal et al., 2013). In this way rumination fuels a downward spiral of low mood.

When practicing mindfulness meditation, a person is asked to intentionally disengage from thoughts of the past or future and to bring awareness to internal or external experiences as they occur in the present moment and to let go of judgments. For example, in breathing meditation, a person is encouraged to notice when his or her mind wanders to thoughts of the past or future, and when this occurs, to let go of these thoughts and redirect his or her attention to the feeling of the breath in the body. Through this process of noticing when and where the mind has wandered, or when judgment is present, then disengaging and redirecting attention (e.g., back to the breath or body), it is postulated that a person learns the skill of disengaging from ruminative cycles of thought. Experimental studies confirm that mindfulness practice is associated with reductions in rumination (Deyo et al., 2009; Jain et al., 2007; Kingston, Dooley, Bates, Lawlor, & Malone, 2007; van der Velden et al., 2015).

Mindfulness interventions can provide an antidote to rumination by teaching the ability to recognize and disengage from the "doing mode of mind," of which rumination is a key example, and instead engage the "being mode of mind" (Kabat-Zinn, 2013; Segal et al., 2013). The doing mode of mind is characterized by problem solving, comparing, planning, and accomplishing goals. These goals could include external goals (e.g., a to-do list of daily tasks) or internal goals (e.g., getting rid of depressed mood, becoming happier). The doing mode often involves thoughts of the past or future, as well as comparisons of one's current situation with an idealized standard of how things should be, along with plans to close the gap between the two.

When one considers the doing mode of mind, whether the doing mode of mind is helpful or unhelpful depends on the context. For example, if a person needs to buy groceries, plan a trip, or decide on a strategy for personal finance, the doing mode of mind is appropriately tasked to navigate these situations, which involve the external world. However, when the doing mode of mind is applied to internal states, such as feelings of loneliness, dissatisfaction, or hopelessness, there are often no easily discernible steps to take to change these feelings, and the doing mode of mind is woefully mismatched for this task. To be clear, it would not be unreasonable to be in a doing mode of mind if the goal is to change the circumstances that may contribute to the feeling states. For example, if someone is feeling chronically lonely, it may be reasonable to set a series of goals for increasing meaningful engagement with others. It would not, however, likely be effective to simply desire greater intimacy and connection with others in the absence of behavioral changes. In this way the doing mode can be skillfully applied to support personal goals involving change and growth.

The being mode of mind is characterized by simply being present and open to what is here in the present (Kabat-Zinn, 2013). In the being mode of mind, thoughts are regarded as passing events in mind and not necessarily true or requiring action (Segal et al., 2013). This perspective also applies to feelings and body sensations, which are regarded with friendliness, curiosity, openness, acceptance, and love (Kabat-Zinn, 2013; Segal et al., 2013; D. J. Siegel, 2007). From this perspective, a person's life is lived entirely in the present moment, and by being more engaged in being mode in the present, rather than being focused on memories of the past or plans for the future, a person often finds greater enjoyment and fulfillment. This is not to suggest that a person should not reflect on the past or plan for the future; these are natural and often very helpful capacities. However, bringing awareness to and reducing the automaticity of these habits is helpful, especially for those with depression. The shift to the being mode, as taught in MBIs, has been theorized to reduce suffering by fostering implicational meaning (i.e., the felt or sensed meaning of an experience), and by allowing these experiences to be processed and integrated into new patterns less associated with distress (Teasdale & Chaskalson, 2011b).

Overgeneralized Autobiographical Memory

Another vulnerability factor for depression is a phenomenon termed *overgeneralized autobiographical memory*, which commonly occurs in the wake of trauma. Overgeneralized autobiographical memory is apparent when people are asked to recount a specific memory from their past in response to a word prompt (e.g., *safe, happy, sad, enjoy*) and instead make a general statement (e.g., "I enjoy reading" rather than "I enjoyed the book about mindfulness I read last week"). Those with a history of trauma are apt to use this strategy, which can be considered a form of avoidance, to blunt memories of stressful situations, including traumatic events (Williams & Barnhofer, 2015). Overgeneralized memory is also more likely if a person is prone to being "captured" by self-referential cues that they then ruminate over, or if they have reduced executive functioning for any reason. Over-generality appears to play a role in maintaining current depressive episodes and confers vulnerability to future episodes of depression in the face of negative life events (Williams & Barnhofer, 2015). Some evidence is accruing that mindfulness training reduces overgeneralized memory (Williams & Barnhofer, 2015), perhaps because cultivating the capacity to be present necessarily makes one more aware of specific details of events happening in the moment, bolstered by an attitude of curiosity and nonjudgmental observation.

Discrepancy Monitoring

Depressive symptoms can also be fueled by unfavorable comparisons between what is desired and what is present. These comparisons can be described in terms of a discrepancy monitor, which continually monitors and compares what is present to an idealized standard of what is desired (Segal et al., 2013). This discrepancy monitor can also fuel the habit of rumination (Segal et al., 2013) and can lead people to perpetually attempt to resolve inconsistencies through problem-solving (Sipe & Eisendrath, 2012). While this can be helpful clear action steps are available, it can be problematic in situations that are more difficult to change (e.g., the nature of one's internal experience). A focus on problem-solving in these situations can increase suffering and perpetuate depression (Sipe & Eisendrath, 2012) in no small part because any benefits from these efforts tend to be short-lived, at best, and are frequently ineffective. In mindfulness practice, a person is asked to notice the habit of comparing. The practice is to see clearly that the mind is generating comparisons and to regard the process with curiosity. At times, it can be helpful to encourage gentle noting of the process, using language such as "Hello old friend, comparing mind," or to simply note "comparing mind" when this habit is present. As a person learns to recognize and disengage from habits of judgment and comparisons, he or she can be asked to notice what thoughts and feelings are present in the moment. As a person brings curiosity and openness to thoughts and feelings that arise in the setting of judgment, it may lead to a shift in understanding as to what underlies the tendency to compare or judge.

Fixed or Fused Thinking and Responding

It has long been recognized that depression is associated with additional various styles of thinking (e.g., all or none, exaggeration or minimization, overpersonalization, arbitrary inference, selective abstraction; Clark & Beck, 1990) that can become fixed or fused such that one fails to recognize that how one is thinking may or may not be accurate or helpful. If such fixed beliefs are negatively biased (e.g., "I didn't get a call back for that job interview because they hated me. I'm such a loser"), and becomes a habitual style of thinking, they can fuel poor mood and behavioral retreat. Similarly, fixed ways of responding to stress or to physical or emotional pain or distress (e.g., "It's not fair, I never catch a break"; "There's no way I can be okay if my back doesn't stop hurting me") can be limiting. Mindfulness practice is theorized to address such thinking by fostering the capacity for decentering, which involves the ability to observe one's thoughts as temporary events in the mind, as opposed to reflections of the self that are necessarily true (Fresco et al., 2007; Safran & Segal, 1990) and overlaps with Shapiro's concept of reperceiving introduced in Chapter 1, this volume.

Decentering refers primarily to a person's relationship to thoughts, but in mindfulness practice the decentered perspective is not limited to thoughts—it also includes feelings, body sensations, and other aspects of experience, such as memories, impulses, sounds, and sights. During mindfulness practice, each of these aspects of experience are regarded as transient events to be noticed with an attitude of openness and curiosity, without attempts to change the experience. In this way, mindfulness practice encompasses experiences of both the mind and body. Also, although the term *decentering* could be construed as a sort of distancing or detachment, in mindfulness practices the attitudinal stance is one of friendliness, openness, and acceptance of experience, including difficult experience, rather than distancing.

An alternate label for decentering that may be helpful is *defusing*, which signals that one's identity is no longer fused with what one thinks or feels. For example, mindfulness may enable someone to step back from the thought "I am damaged goods" and notice with compassion that "right now, I'm having the thought that I'm damaged and that doesn't mean I am truly damaged" rather than believing the thought to be true. Thus, a person is encouraged to feel what she or he is feeling—even if is difficult—aided by an attitude of gentleness, kindness, and curiosity. As these abilities are strengthened, it can lead to a greater ability to deal with difficult thoughts, emotions and impulses.

Metacognitive awareness is another term that is closely related to this concept of decentering; it refers to the capacity to recognize depressive thinking in a broader field of awareness (i.e., to be aware that one's experiences are not defined by and confined to these painful thoughts and feelings). The shift in perspective, or reperceiving and stepping back from one's thought process to observe it, as it is learned through mindfulness teaches people the ability to see depressive styles of thinking as characteristic of depression, not of themselves. Through mindfulness training, individuals can learn the ability to see that "these thoughts and feelings aren't me" (Allen, Bromley, Kuyken, & Sonnenberg, 2009). When working with depressive symptoms in clinical practice, mindfulness teachers can reframe reports of depressive symptoms by asking participants to simply note "sad thoughts are here," or "greetings, old friend depression," rather than using language that denotes fusing or identifying with the symptoms such as "I am depressed" or "my depression symptoms."

In addition to decentering, the development of self-compassion appears to play a key role that facilitates a shift to a decentered or metacognitive perspective. In a study comparing mindfulness-based cognitive therapy (MBCT) to maintenance antidepressants, individuals who developed greater self-compassion uncoupled the relationship between depressive styles of thinking and symptoms of depression (Kuyken et al., 2010). In other words, dysfunctional thinking styles were not necessarily reduced, but for people who developed self-compassion during MBCT there was a change in the relationship between cognitive reactivity (i.e., beliefs, assumptions, and rules considered dysfunctional that are usually associated with depressive-style thinking) and depressive symptoms. The moderation of depressive symptoms at 15 months follow-up as it relates to change in self-compassion during MBCT is illustrated in Figure 2.1. In the figure, cognitive reactivity is represented on the *x*-axis. Cognitive reactivity was measured after the 8-week MBCT course and is defined as the change in dysfunctional attitudes before and after a sad mood induction. The Self-Compassion Scale (SCS) change represents the change in self-compassion over the course of MBCT, and the *y*-axis represents depressive symptoms at 15 months follow-up. This figure demonstrates that for patients who had a depressive-style of thinking induced by a sad mood (i.e., had high cognitive reactivity) after completing MBCT, that there was not an associated increase in depressive symptoms 15 months later *if* they had an increase in self-compassion during the course of MBCT. These findings suggest that although negative patterns of thinking may persist or reappear after participation in a mindfulness intervention, what matters for depressive outcome is how one responds to these negative thought patterns (e.g., with or without self-compassion).

Mindfulness and Depression: The Evidence

There is a robust literature evaluating MBIs among individuals with current depressive symptoms as well as among individuals with a prior history of major depression not currently depressed but at high risk of a depressive

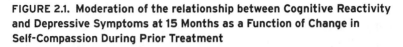

FIGURE 2.1. Moderation of the relationship between Cognitive Reactivity and Depressive Symptoms at 15 Months as a Function of Change in Self-Compassion During Prior Treatment

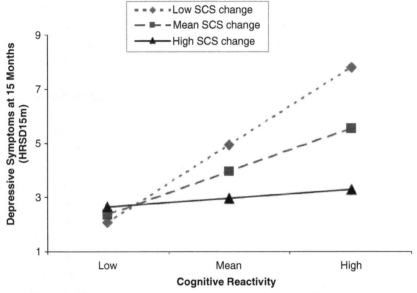

From "How Does Mindfulness-Based Cognitive Therapy Work?," by W. Kuyken, E. Watkins, E. Holden, K. White, R. S. Taylor, S. Byford, A. Evans, S. Radford, J. D. Teasdale, and T. Dalgleish, 2010, *Behaviour Research and Therapy*, *48*, p. 1111. Copyright 2010 by Elsevier. Adapted with permission.

relapse; there are nearly 50 published randomized clinical trials (RCTs) to draw upon (Goldberg et al., 2018). However, although depression commonly occurs following trauma, the extant literature on outcomes of MBIs has generally not been conducted in the setting of trauma. (Findings on depressive symptoms in RCTs evaluating MBIs for PTSD are noted in Chapter 1 with regard to the Polusny et al. [2015] and L. L. Davis et al. [2018] studies.)

Many of the trials evaluating outcomes for depression studied MBCT, which was adapted from MBSR to prevent relapse of depression (Segal et al., 2013). For this reason, it is helpful to understand the differences between MBSR and MBCT. Overall, MBSR and MBCT are very similar; the differences in curriculum account for only a small portion of class time. MBCT is a manualized 8-week program delivered in groups that are typically smaller than MBSR (up to 12 participants, whereas MBSR may have 20& participants), with slightly shorter class sessions than MBSR (2 hours per class for MBCT rather than 2.5 hours for MBSR; Segal et al., 2013). MBCT is typically coded as therapy, whereas MBSR is typically coded as group education.

Just as in MBSR, each MBCT class session emphasizes instruction in mindfulness meditation (e.g., breathing meditation, body scan meditation, gentle yoga, walking meditation) and provides opportunities to engage in group discussions. In MBCT, elements of cognitive behavior therapy relevant to depression, such as imagining specific scenarios and noting thoughts that arise, as a means of drawing attention to depressive styles of thinking, are also incorporated. Psychoeducation about specific mechanisms of depressive relapse is also provided in MBCT, whereas in MBSR education about the stress response along with general education about styles of distorted thinking is usually included.

MBCT was originally developed to prevent relapse of major depression (i.e., to prevent individuals with a history of major depressive episodes who are not currently depressed from experiencing additional depressive episodes; Segal et al., 2013). Clinical trials indicate that MBCT markedly reduces the rate of depressive relapse (see below), and initial evidence supports a positive impact of MBCT on other conditions, including pain, fatigue, PTSD, and current depressive symptoms (Eisendrath et al., 2015; Hofmann et al., 2010; King et al., 2013; Lakhan & Schofield, 2013; Moore & Martin, 2015; Rimes & Wingrove, 2013; Sipe & Eisendrath, 2012).

Depression Relapse

We discuss MBIs for prevention of relapse of major depression before addressing mindfulness for current depressive symptoms because the research base is significantly stronger for relapse prevention. Multiple high-quality RCTs have evaluated whether MBCT prevents depressive relapse, and in a meta-analysis of six RCTs (N 8 593 patients) MBCT was found to reduce the rate of depressive relapse (relative risk reduction of 43%) compared with treatment as usual (TAU) or placebo for people with three or more prior episodes of depression (Piet & Hougaard, 2011). Another more recent meta-analysis included data from nine RCTs (N 8 1,258 patients) and found that MBCT was associated with a reduced risk of depressive relapse (hazard ratio 0.69) over a 60-week follow-up period compared with all non-MBCT treatments (e.g., usual care, antidepressants, psychoeducation; Kuyken et al., 2016). Patients with more severe depression at baseline received greater benefit from MBCT compared with non-MBCT treatments, and age or sex were not predictive of outcomes.

In the Piet and Hougaard (2011) meta-analysis, a significant reduction in rate of depressive relapse was limited to individuals with three or more prior episodes of major depression. The influence of number of prior depressive episodes on outcomes of MBCT (Piet & Hougaard, 2011) is postulated to occur because different mechanisms may cause depressive relapse for individuals with two or fewer episodes as compared with those with multiple episodes of depression. Those with two or fewer prior episodes of depression may be more likely to experience depressive relapse because of external events, whereas those with three or more prior relapses may be more likely to have their relapses triggered by autonomous ruminative cycles, which are effectively targeted by MBCT (Ma & Teasdale, 2004).

The marked reduction in rate of depressive relapse for those with three or more prior episodes of major depression is illustrated in Figure 2.2 by

FIGURE 2.2. Survival (Nonrelapse/Nonrecurrence) Curves Comparing Relapse/ Recurrence to *Diagnostic and Statistical Manual of Mental Disorders* (4th ed.) Major Depression for Treatment-as-Usual (TAU) and MBCT in Patients With Three or More Previous Episodes of Major Depression (Intent-to-Treat Sample)

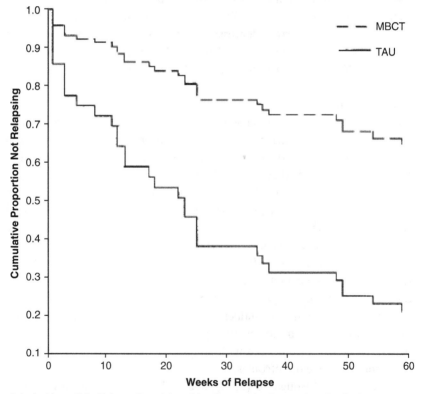

Adapted from "Mindfulness-Based Cognitive Therapy for Depression: Replication and Exploration of Differential Relapse Prevention Effects," by S. H. Ma and J. D. Teasdale, 2004, *Journal of Consulting and Clinical Psychology*, 72, p. 36. Copyright 2004 by the American Psychological Association.

findings from one key trial (Ma & Teasdale, 2004). In this trial, patients currently in remission from major depression were randomly assigned to MBCT or TAU and followed for 1 year at 3-month intervals. Figure 2.2 illustrates the rate of relapse of depression in an intent-to-treat analysis for those with a prior history of three or more prior episodes of depressive episodes before entering the trial. The figure shows that the cumulative proportion not relapsing was significantly higher among those randomly assigned to MBCT.

Although the above studies provide convincing evidence that MBCT is superior to usual care, the trials were not designed to directly compare MBCT with the current standard of care for prevention of depressive relapse: maintenance antidepressants (though a subset of usual care patients in the above studies received antidepressants). In the Kuyken et al. (2016) meta-analysis, when limited to four RCTs in which maintenance antidepressants were compared with MBCT, over a 60-week follow-up period there was a reduced risk of depressive relapse for those assigned to MBCT, with a hazard ratio 0.77 (0.60–0.98; Kuyken et al., 2016). In the largest individual trial (included in the Kuyken et al., 2016, meta-analysis), which was a well-designed, single-blinded multicenter RCT with 24-month follow-up involving 424 patients, both interventions had similar positive outcomes in terms of prevention of depressive relapse, quality of life, and residual depressive symptoms (Kuyken et al., 2015). There was no evidence that MBCT was superior to maintenance antidepressants. The proportion of people without relapse of major depression who were randomly assigned to maintenance antidepressant medications (mADM) or MBCT are shown in Figure 2.3.

An additional question is whether the combination of MBCT plus continued antidepressants is superior to MBCT followed by tapering of antidepressants. A clinical trial (*N* 8 249) addressed this question by comparing MBCT with discontinuation of mADM to the combination of MBCT plus mADM; the goal of the study was to determine whether patients who underwent MBCT could safely withdraw antidepressants. The results indicated that those assigned to withdraw antidepressants after MBCT were more likely to experience depressive relapse as compared with MBCT with continued mADM (Huijbers et al., 2016).

Overall, the literature indicates that MBCT produces outcomes similar to maintenance antidepressants for prevention of depressive relapse, but a strategy of both MBCT and maintenance antidepressants is likely optimal (Creswell, 2017). On the basis of the above evidence, the National Health Service (NHS) in the United Kingdom recommended that MBCT

FIGURE 2.3. Survival Cures (of Not Relapse or Recurrence) Over a 24-Month Follow-up Period for the Intention-to-Treat Population

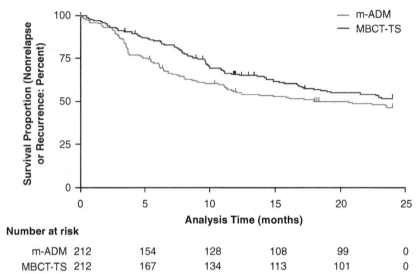

Number at risk

m-ADM	212	154	128	108	99	0
MBCT-TS	212	167	134	113	101	0

mADM = maintenance antidepressant medication. MBCT-TS = mindfulness-based cognitive therapy with support to taper or discontinue antidepressant medication. Adapted from "Effectiveness and Cost-Effectiveness of Mindfulness-Based Cognitive Therapy Compared With Maintenance Antidepressant Treatment in the Prevention of Depressive Relapse or Recurrence (PREVENT): A Randomised Controlled Trial," by W. Kuyken, R. Hayes, B. Barrett, R. Byng, T. Dalgleish, D. Kessler, . . . S. Byford, 2015, *The Lancet, 386,* p. 69. CC BY.

undergo broad implementation as standard care for prevention of depressive relapse (Crane & Kuyken, 2013; Mindfulness All-Party Parliamentary Group, 2015).

In the broader literature encompassing all MBIs (i.e., those not limited to MBCT), Goldberg et al. (2018) performed a large systematic review and meta-analysis and identified 49 RCTs evaluating an MBI for either acute depression or prevention of depressive relapse, 30 of which compared an MBI with no treatment, nine of which compared an MBI with a specific active comparison condition, and 10 of which compared an MBI with an evidence-based treatment (EBT). At the end of treatment, when compared with those assigned to no treatment, those receiving an MBI showed significantly better depression outcomes (either reducing acute depression or preventing relapse), while the comparisons involving specific active control conditions showed more modest but still statistically significant advantage for people assigned to an MBI. Across the trials comparing MBIs and EBTs, there were no differences in depressive outcomes detected at the end of treatment. This basic pattern of findings was also apparent in the meta-analytic models involving the 25 studies with longer follow-up assessments such that MBIs outperformed no treatment and specific active controls but showed similar depression outcomes to EBTs.

Current Depression

To evaluate whether the strong evidence supporting the effect of MBCT on preventing relapse of major depression is apparent for those with current depression, Goldberg et al. (2018) performed a meta-analysis of RCTs assessing outcomes of MBCT for this group of patients (Goldberg et al., 2019). Across the 13 included studies (N 8 1,046), comparison conditions were categorized as either nonspecific or specific, where the former referred to attention placebo conditions, TAU, or no treatment, and the latter included actual therapies meant to address depression symptoms. The results indicated that at the end of treatment people assigned to MBCT had better depression outcomes than those assigned to a nonspecific control condition, though this benefit was not maintained at the longest follow-up. Across studies comparing MBCT to a specific comparator meant to address depression, no differences between groups were found either at the end of treatment or the longest follow-up (Goldberg et al., 2019). Overall, the results at posttreatment indicated that patients currently experiencing depressive symptoms respond to MBCT with moderate effect sizes compared with nonspecific controls but did not outperform other therapies meant to address depression. Also, at longest follow-up, MBCT did not continue to out-perform nonspecific or specific control conditions. These findings support the use of MBCT for patients with current depressive symptoms, although additional research is needed to clarify long-term outcomes.

We close this discussion of MBIs for depression with an overview of recent efforts to ascertain the mechanisms of change associated with receipt of an MBI. Understanding mechanisms of change associated with a specific intervention can help refine the intervention to improve upon the key elements leading to salutary change (Kazdin & Nock, 2003; Kraemer, Wilson, Fairburn, & Agras, 2002). To evaluate the mechanisms of behavior change associated with MBCT in the context of recurrent major depression, van der Velden et al. (2015) undertook a systematic review of 23 studies based on 17 trials. Although all but three of the studies were RCTs, as the review authors pointed out, most of the trials were not designed to rigorously evaluate mechanisms of behavior change (see Kazdin & Nock, 2003, and

Nock, 2007, for an overview of the criteria for establishing a mechanism of behavior change). This fundamental limitation of the literature notwithstanding, the review found that increased mindfulness, self-compassion, and meta-awareness as well as decreased rumination and worry were associated with improved depression outcomes in the majority of studies examining these factors. These findings are in line with the predominant ideas reviewed above regarding how MBIs likely exert their effects on depression.

SUBSTANCE USE DISORDERS

It has long been recognized that individuals with PTSD are at substantially elevated risk relative to those without PTSD of developing problems with alcohol and other drugs and to smoke cigarettes (Goldstein et al., 2016). Although there is some evidence to support other theories regarding the relationship between PTSD and substance use issues, the self-medication theory is the most widely studied and has the most support (Simpson, Stappenbeck, Luterek, Lehavot, & Kaysen, 2014). The self-medication theory posits that individuals may come to rely on alcohol, tobacco, or other drugs to cope with the distress and negative affect associated with PTSD and any additional co-occurring psychiatric conditions (Khantzian, 2003). Over time, reliance on substances to deal with emotional (and physical) discomfort can cause other coping strategies to atrophy and can lead to an automaticity that is essentially the antithesis of mindfulness (Garland & Howard, 2018). Complicating the clinical picture further, heavy use of substances over extended periods of time can lead to tolerance of the substances such that more is needed to achieve the same effects and physiological dependence on the substances such that people need to ingest them to feel "normal." In addition, the accrual of life consequences resulting from behaviors associated with substance abuse can add additional stress and strain, which can potentially lead to increased desire to use substances to cope. It is no doubt easy to see how people can become caught in a vicious cycle as they attempt to chase relief through use of substances that often come with additional sets of problems.

Mindfulness and Pathways of Change for Substance Abuse

Low stress tolerance (Koob & Volkow, 2010; Sinha, 2007) and automatic responses to people, places, and things are associated with substance use and can make it difficult for individuals with addictions to change habit patterns associated with problematic use (Garland & Howard, 2018).

Additionally, overreliance on alcohol and drugs can lead to a lack of salience for situations and experiences that are not tied to substances so that little else is able to match the intensity and the immediate gratification derived from substance use, thereby further reinforcing use patterns and atrophying less harmful reinforcers (Garland & Howard, 2018).

Although still in its infancy, a clinical trials literature is developing that has begun to evaluate mechanisms of behavior change associated with MBIs for people with substance use problems. These studies have not specifically included individuals with co-occurring PTSD and substance use problems and do not address comorbidities generally, but understanding the potential ways that mindfulness may help to alleviate substance use problems is useful foundational knowledge that it likely relevant in the context of comorbidities, including with PTSD. Preliminary evidence suggests that increases in aspects of mindfulness such as acceptance, awareness, and nonjudgment mediate the effects of MBIs on craving and substance use (Garland & Howard, 2018). Decreases in stress reactivity and improvement in stress recovery as well as decreased reactivity to cravings and substance use cues have also been found to be associated with mindfulness training and in turn are associated with decreased substance craving and use (Bowen et al., 2014). Overall, there is growing evidence that suggests participation in MBIs may assist people struggling with addictions to decouple their thoughts and feelings, including cravings, from substance use itself (Li, Howard, Garland, McGovern, & Lazar, 2017).

Mindfulness training may also help people with substance use problems develop metacognition, which, as noted above, refers to the ability to step back and observe one's own thinking process rather than allowing one's thoughts and impulses to run unmonitored (Garland & Howard, 2018). This process of stepping back allows a person to recognize that there is more going on within oneself and in the larger environment than the distress felt in the moment. This process of stepping back can enable people to see beyond the immediate desire for relief so they can make deliberate choices that may be more in keeping with their values (Bowen et al., 2014). A participant in one of our own MBI groups reported that learning mindfulness gave him the ability to make different choices:

> Something to help me make proper decisions when I'm dealing with a stressful situation, and when the depression kicks in to make just smarter choices rather than picking up the bottle again, because that's been my escape in the past and obviously it doesn't work.

Another pathway through which MBIs are hypothesized to reduce substance use is by increasing the ability to experience natural rewards or by increasing the appreciation of rewards not obtained through substance use, which Garland and Howard (2018) called "the restructuring reward hypothesis." According to this hypothesis, MBIs hold the potential to shift the focus from rewards obtained by substances back to natural rewards that may have been available to the person before substance misuse took hold. In mindfulness, this is taught by increasing awareness and appreciation through savoring of pleasant experiences in daily life. For example, many MBIs teach mindful eating, in which a person is taught to savor the experience of eating food. In theory, increasing natural reward processing holds the potential to reduce cravings and addictive behavior; and there is some evidence in support of this (Garland & Howard, 2018).

The overarching goals of MBIs for substance use disorders are to increase capacity for present-moment awareness and to help people increase their capacity to tolerate and accept the painful thoughts and feelings that will inevitably arise as part of the human condition without the need to self-medicate them with alcohol and drugs. Mindfulness also holds the potential to increase the appreciation of rewards that occur naturally in life, which can shift the focus away from rewards obtained by substances.

Evidence for Mindfulness Interventions for Substance Use Problems

Relative to the literature on MBIs for depression and depressive relapse, the literature on MBIs for addictions and smoking is much sparser, with a total of only 16 RCTs available to date (Goldberg et al., 2018). Across the five studies comparing an MBI for addiction to no treatment, Goldberg and colleagues did not find a significant difference in outcomes between conditions at the end of treatment (none of the studies had a longer follow-up assessment). However, in the RCTs involving a specific active control condition, there was a modest effect in favor of the MBIs at the end of treatment across the seven addiction studies, but this advantage was not maintained across the four studies with a longer follow-up period. Across the four studies comparing an MBI to an EBT for smoking there was a moderate effect favoring the MBIs, though there were not sufficient data at longer follow-up intervals to determine whether this advantage for MBIs holds up over time. (There are currently no MBI vs. evidence-based therapy RCTs addressing addiction other than to cigarette smoking.) These findings echo an earlier systematic review and meta-analysis of MBIs for addiction conducted by Li et al. (2017), although the older review did not account for the quality of the comparison conditions as Goldberg et al. did (Chiesa & Serretti, 2014; Goldberg et al., 2018). Overall, the available evidence suggests that MBIs may have some utility in the treatment of substance use disorders, but further refinements or augmentations are likely needed to address their waning effectiveness at longer follow-ups.

CHRONIC PAIN AND OTHER SOMATIC CONDITIONS

Trauma increases the risk of developing a chronic physical pain syndrome, including low back pain, chronic pelvic pain, headaches, fibromyalgia, chronic regional and widespread pain, orofacial pain, and self-reported arthritis (R. D. Siegel, 2015). Those with a history of abusive childhoods appear particularly vulnerable to developing a pain syndrome (D. A. Davis, Luecken, & Zautra, 2005). As a result, many people with PTSD must simultaneously cope with both PTSD symptoms and chronic pain. For this reason, when working with people with a history of trauma, it is helpful for the group leader or therapist to have a working knowledge of how mindfulness techniques can be applied to chronic pain.

Chronic Pain

Dealing with multiple conditions and life difficulties can be stressful, and increased stress tends to worsen the clinical course of chronic pain, as does the presence of psychiatric conditions such as PTSD or depression (Beck & Clapp, 2011; Day, 2017; Kroenke et al., 2011; Otis et al., 2010). Decades of research have made it clear that psychological processes play important roles in chronic pain by influencing central sensitization, making it more likely that acute pain becomes chronic, and shaping the way in which pain is interpreted (Day, 2017). Given that psychological factors have a strong effect on the clinical course of pain, they represent ideal targets for clinical interventions, and CBT-based approaches are widely accepted as the gold standard approach. However, as is the case for PTSD, not all people with chronic pain respond to CBT, and not all people prefer CBT as a therapeutic approach. MBIs are another option for treatment for chronic pain.

In the next subsections, we provide an overview of the mechanisms through which mindfulness practice can benefit people with chronic pain, and review the literature on clinical outcomes of MBIs for chronic pain. Additional suggestions about how to effectively teach specific mindfulness practice to people with chronic pain are provided in Chapter 4.

Mindfulness and Pathways of Change for Chronic Pain

There are multiple pathways by which a person who has experienced trauma is predisposed to develop chronic pain. One important factor is the tendency following trauma to interpret ambiguous stimuli as dangerous or threatening, which leads to autonomic arousal (Pole et al., 2007; R. D. Siegel, 2015). The tendency to interpret pain as threatening (known as pain catastrophizing) can lead to fear of future pain (Vlaeyen & Linton, 2000). Paradoxically, as a result of fear and catastrophizing, a vicious cycle can be established whereby fear of pain results in hypersensitivity to pain, increased muscle tension and disuse of the painful area, which in turn leads to loss of strength and flexibility, and predisposes to future injury (R. D. Siegel, 2015; Vlaeyen & Linton, 2000).

The tendency to interpret bodily sensations as potentially threatening is considered a form of hypervigilance as applied to bodily sensations rather than the external world. People who develop chronic pain syndromes often also develop beliefs that bodily sensations mean the body is damaged, which can further contribute to fear of movement. For example, a person may hold beliefs about whether he is able to participate in certain activities because of chronic pain, including the activities proposed in MBIs, such as periods of sitting, walking, or stretching. These factors can present clinically as catastrophizing, anxiety sensitivity, and avoidant coping, which in turn lead to stress-related nervous system changes (Beck & Clapp, 2011). Depression, pain catastrophizing, and anxiety are correlated with worse pain severity and disability in cross-sectional studies; longitudinal studies show that when these factors decrease, pain severity and disability improve (Bair et al., 2013; Campbell et al., 2012; Lucey et al., 2011; Scott, Kroenke, Wu, & Yu, 2016).

Jensen (2011) posited that MBIs provide benefit in the context of chronic pain through one or more of the following pathways: (a) environmental/social variables, (b) brain states, (c) cognitive content, (d) cognitive processes/ coping, and (e) behavior. An evidence-based theoretical model of MBIs for chronic pain by Day, Jensen, Ehde, and Thorn (2014) builds on these ideas and shows that MBIs favorably influence each of these five factors, and in addition positively influence a sixth factor: emotion and affect. In this empirically derived model, mindfulness practices are considered to be forms of exposure that lead to change by uncoupling the sensory and cognitive– evaluative networks, reducing pain catastrophizing, changing pain beliefs, increasing pain acceptance, improving approach-oriented coping, and bettering positive affect and emotion regulation (Day et al., 2014). We now provide additional commentary, based primarily on our clinical experience, as further explanation of how MBIs may be applied to the mechanism of change described previously.

The overarching theme of self-care, whether it be managing stress more effectively or bringing attention to how our minds are functioning, is emphasized in MBIs and is often very helpful to those with chronic pain. MBIs emphasize changing the relationship to pain and learning to practice greater self-care, whether by more effectively managing stress or by learning that one's sense of well-being or symptoms are helped by simply slowing down. The theme of self-care came through in an interview with a woman who participated in an MBI at our site. She summarized how an MBI helped her pain as

> it's given me a different relationship in terms of pain. I'm able to see it in a different light that pushing through and dragging on is not always the right answer. . . . Which was the opposite of the way my brain was working on it.

As described by this patient, the focus of MBIs for chronic pain is learning to relate to a difficult experience—chronic pain—in a new way, which can lead to increased functionality. MBIs do not directly focus on attempting to reduce pain severity, although that might occur as a person becomes less physiologically reactive to pain (R. D. Siegel, 2015). In MBIs, the focus is on teaching people the skill of noticing and disengaging from layers of reactivity to the experience of chronic pain.

A fundamental teaching point of MBIs is to notice patterns of automatic thinking, including noticing the tendency to catastrophize or ruminate. As a way of working with catastrophizing in MBIs, a person is asked to notice that physical sensations of pain or discomfort are distinct from associated thoughts and emotions. Learning to distinguish the sensory component from the affective and cognitive components of pain can lead to an uncoupling of the cognitive elements and emotional elements from the sensory experience, and this uncoupling can provide a newfound opportunity to work with troubling thoughts and emotions. It is this uncoupling that is theorized to result in improved regulation of affect and behavioral change (Kabat-Zinn, 1982). Central to these salutatory changes is the cultivation of increased moment-to-moment contact with what is actually happening in the here and now. This exposure to the present moment is thought to allow people to distinguish what they fear from what they are actually experiencing.

Accordingly, the concept that thoughts are passing events in the mind, which may or may not represent reality, is introduced in MBIs and can be particularly helpful when applied to thoughts and beliefs surrounding chronic pain. In MBIs, the practice is to hold these thoughts in a broader field of awareness, to note the thoughts as passing mental events, and to recognize that ideas or beliefs may or may not represent reality. In MBIs, a person learns experientially that thoughts are thoughts, which may or may not be true. MBIs also include material designed to increase the awareness of thoughts, emotions, and sensations related to pleasant and unpleasant events as well as how habitual judgments about them can lead to reactivity and catastrophizing (e.g., "I can't stand another day of this pain"). By engaging repeatedly in mindfulness meditation practices that encourage openness and curiosity rather than tightness and judgment, class participants can learn to notice their habitual reactive responses and return to their breath. As an example, a person may understandably be afraid of injury and believe that she is unable to participate in the movement practices included in MBIs (e.g., gentle yoga in MBSR). During class sessions, a person is encouraged to regard such fears and thoughts with openness and curiosity, and to gently move forward with these practices to the best of her ability. It is important to note that this often involves significant modifications, and that people should be simultaneously encouraged to trust their own limitations and opt out if they think it is the wisest course of action. For movement practices in particular, gently practicing movement in MBIs is theorized to lead to reductions in fear of movement or fear of pain or reinjury, which are key components in the disability associated with chronic pain (Day, 2017).

The comments in this section are intended to provide both a practical and a conceptual framework for understanding how MBIs can lead to improved outcomes for chronic pain. Additional practical suggestions for teaching specific practices to people with chronic pain are provided in Chapters 3 and 4.

Evidence for MBIs for Chronic Pain

In a recent meta-analysis, Goldberg et al. (2018) identified 33 pain trials, 24 of which compared an MBI with no treatment and nine of which compared an MBI with a specific active control condition that accounted for factors like time and attention from a therapist or instructor (Goldberg et al., 2018). When compared with no treatment, a moderate effect favoring MBIs was found immediately after treatment ended (d 8 .45; 0.30 (0.60), while there was no appreciable difference found when MBIs for pain were compared to specific active control conditions. This same pattern of findings was seen across the 30 pain studies that included a longer follow-up period (Goldberg et al., 2018). A systematic review of MBIs by Creswell (2017) highlights four recent RCTs comparing MBIs with active control conditions for individuals with chronic pain; in three of the studies the MBIs had superior outcomes, while in one the MBI had better outcomes than the TAU condition and comparable outcomes to a robust, matched CBT for pain program (Creswell, 2017). Other systematic reviews also reported that participation in mindfulness programs is associated with reduced pain intensity (Reiner et al., 2013), reduced symptom severity (Lakhan & Schofield, 2013), and reduced depressive symptoms associated with pain (Veehof, Oskam, Schreurs, & Bohlmeijer, 2011). An additional systematic review found benefit of MBSR for chronic low back pain (Skelly et al., 2018). Overall, these findings indicate that MBIs can be considered viable treatment options for those suffering from chronic pain, but additional high-quality research is needed.

Functional Somatic Syndromes

Functional somatic syndromes, also referred to as medically unexplained symptoms, are among the most common reasons people seek medical care (Afari et al., 2014; Burton, 2003). A consistent feature across functional somatic syndromes is that they occur in excess among people who have sustained trauma; findings from a meta-analysis of 71 studies indicated that persons exposed to trauma were 2.7 times more likely to develop a functional somatic syndrome (Afari et al., 2014). Functional somatic syndromes are chronic symptom-based syndromes for which no organic pathology can be demonstrated (Burton, 2003); examples include fibromyalgia, temporomandibular disorder, and IBS. These syndromes commonly overlap such that many patients meet criteria for more than one functional somatic syndrome (Wessely, Nimnuan, & Sharpe, 1999).

One of the most common functional syndromes is IBS, which commonly co-occurs with PTSD (Dobie et al., 2004; Maguen, Madden, Cohen, Bertenthal, & Seal, 2014). IBS is characterized by recurrent abdominal pain that is related to defecation and associated with a change in stool frequency or a change in the form of stool (Lacy & Patel, 2017). Clinically, individuals with IBS often have significant reductions in quality of life (Addante et al., 2018), and chronic life stress is the main predictor of IBS symptom severity (Drossman et al., 2000). In addition, IBS patients demonstrate reduced thresholds to report pain, which is attributed to symptom hypervigilance (Drossman, 2016). Other potentially modifiable factors that play a role in IBS clinical outcomes include anxiety about gastrointestinal symptoms, beliefs about the meaning of symptoms, catastrophizing, and perceived lack of social support. These factors play important roles in influencing medication use, health care visits, costs, and disability for IBS patients (Drossman, 2016; Van Oudenhove et al., 2016).

As is apparent from the foregoing discussion, psychological processes play a key role in the clinical course of IBS, and this has led to studies of MBIs to treat this condition (Thakur et al., 2018). Though the literature base regarding MBIs as treatment for IBS is much smaller than that for pain, findings to date suggest they hold some promise for this condition. One meta-analysis of three RCTs (Lakhan & Schofield, 2013) and another meta-analysis of six RCTs of MBIs for IBS both found evidence of improved symptoms. Another systematic review of MBSR for physical conditions found preliminary evidence suggesting that MBSR improves IBS (Crowe et al., 2016). A before-and-after study of individuals with both PTSD and IBS at baseline found that only 40% still met IBS criteria 4 months after completing MBSR (Harding, Simpson, & Kearney, 2018). Additional studies are needed, and although a history of trauma is common among patients with IBS, to date none of the RCTs specifically assessed individuals with comorbid PTSD and IBS.

Fibromyalgia is characterized by generalized pain involving multiple body regions, lasting for at least 3 months and meeting specific criteria for severity (Wolfe et al., 2016). Associated psychological features often include depression, catastrophizing, and sleep disturbances. A recent review identified two trials of MBSR for fibromyalgia, each of which lacked long-term follow-up (Skelly et al., 2018). No clear short-term benefits were seen for measures of functionality, pain, depression, anxiety, sleep, or fatigue for patients randomized to MBSR as compared with either a waitlist control or attention control (education/relaxation/stretching) in two trials. A third trial involved a small of individuals with fibromyalgia (*N* 8 32) and randomized them to either a MBI or a waitlist control and found lower levels of anger, anxiety, and depression among those assigned to the MBI (Amutio, Franco, Pérez-Fuentes, Gázquez, & Mercader, 2015). The same research group also reported improved sleep for fibromyalgia patients who participate in an MBI as compared with waitlist control (Amutio et al., 2018). A noninterventional study examined the relationship between mindfulness and psychological factors for patients with fibromyalgia and found that the association between catastrophizing and pain intensity was moderated by facets of mindfulness (Dorado et al., 2018). Additional study of MBIs as treatment for fibromyalgia is needed.

Does Participation in an MBI Result in Improvement in Multiple Diagnoses?

Up to this point, we have considered the literature on clinical outcomes for individual diagnoses. But as we have discussed, given that comorbidity is the norm and not the exception among trauma survivors, does improvement across multiple conditions occur following participation in an MBI? In theory, if people can learn to recognize habits (e.g., avoidance, rumination, catastrophizing, fixed or fused styles of thinking) in one or more areas of their lives, and if they learn instead to respond mindfully, they can begin to apply this new way of responding to a diverse range of challenges. This may result in benefit across conditions because, as described in this and the prior chapter, several of the mechanisms that mindfulness is posited to impact are known to maintain or worsen symptoms for multiple post-trauma sequelae. Although these have been incompletely studied, there is some evidence that teaching MBSR does benefit trauma survivors across multiple conditions. For example, the Polusny et al. (2015) RCT showed greater improvements for both PTSD and depression for MBSR as compared with an active control; chronic pain and substance misuse were not measured. In our own work, we performed a small RCT that compared MBSR plus usual care with usual care only for veterans with Gulf War illness, which is characterized by unexplained chronic pain, fatigue, depression, and attention disturbances (N 8 55), of whom 82% also met criteria for probable PTSD. Among those with PTSD at baseline, significantly greater reductions in PTSD symptoms occurred over time in the MBSR arm as compared with usual care at the immediate post-MBSR time point. At 6-month follow-up, improvements in PTSD were maintained at the level of a statistical trend (p 8 .08). In terms of other symptoms, those randomized to MBSR also had significant improvements at 6-month follow-up in measures of pain, fatigue, depression, and self-reported attention/memory lapses, with medium-to-large effect sizes (Kearney et al., 2016). These findings provide initial support for the possibility that MBSR can simultaneously benefit multiple clinical conditions, using the standard MBSR format and as taught by instructors with an understanding of relevant clinical conditions. The main findings are summarized in Figure 2.4, which shows change in five outcomes over time for those randomized to MBSR or TAU.

SUMMARY

Because it can be difficult to conceptualize how these various trauma-related issues can inform and compound one another in the lives of real individuals, we close this chapter with a brief case history that illustrates both the burden of multiple comorbidities and how mindfulness training can be helpful in ameliorating the attendant issues and symptoms.

Mr. H is a 62-year-old non-Hispanic White man who has been married for 30 years. He developed PTSD after an on-the-job back injury, which left him unable to work. After surgery to fuse damaged vertebra in his spine, he dealt with debilitating chronic pain as well as significant depression and passive thoughts about suicide (e.g., thinking it would be ok if he were hit by a bus or if lightning struck him). He remained clear, however, that he would not want to hurt his family by deliberately harming himself.

FIGURE 2.4. Outcomes Over Time for Mindfulness-based Stress Reduction Compared with Treatment as Usual for Veterans With Gulf War Illness (Intention-to-Treat Analysis)

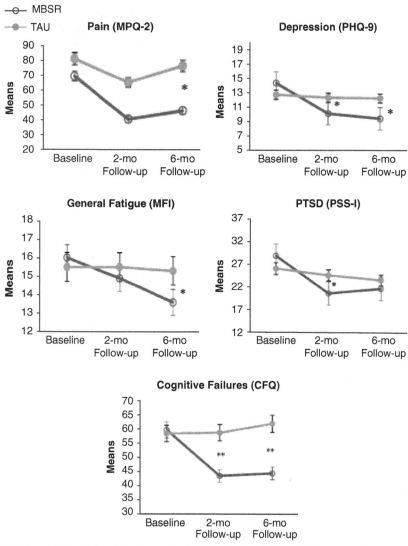

CFQ 8 Cognitive Failure Questionnaire; MFI 8 Multidimensional Fatigue Inventory; MPQ-2 8 McGill Pain Questionnaire 2; PHQ-9 8 Patient Health Questionnaire; PSS-1 8 PTSD Symptom Scale Interview; PTSD 8 posttraumatic stress disorder. *p } .05, **p } .01 for significance of group ° time interaction. From "Mindfulness-Based Stress Reduction in Addition to Usual Care Is Associated With Improvements in Pain, Fatigue, and Cognitive Failures Among Veterans With Gulf War Illness," by D. J. Kearney, T. L. Simpson, C. A Malte, B. Felleman, M. E. Martinez, and S. C. Hunt, 2016, *The American Journal of Medicine*, 129, p. 211. Copyright 2016 by Elsevier. Adapted with permission.

Mr. H drank heavily several times a week to cope when he felt overwhelmed by physical pain, PTSD symptoms, and his current circumstances. Historically, Mr. H recalled his father having used harsh corporal punishment frequently and having gotten the message from both his parents that he was not as smart as his siblings and that he was lazy. For years after the accident he got feedback from his family that he was short-tempered and hard to be around.

Mr. H was referred to MBSR by his primary care provider. Although he expressed some skepticism and initially thought his provider was implying his pain was all in his head, he was assured this was not the case and decided it would be worth giving mindfulness training a try as an adjunct to his other treatments. When interviewed about his experience with MBSR about 6 months after the group Mr. H said,

> Because I have chronic back pain I was thoroughly convinced that I can only bend so far, I can only move a certain way, and so I had this thought process that said you should know I can't do that. You should know that we can't do this.

However, he shared that

> when I started doing the stretching and other exercises, I saw I could actually move around, so I joined the gym. Because of that, I go to the gym every morning at six o'clock now, and do stretching and stuff like that.

Additionally, he said he learned "to slow down and think things through. Just deal with things going on right now" and noted

> My wife said I got a lot calmer. I actually felt like . . . I slowed down because of my meditation. I have a mind that never cuts off. . . . I was having anxiety so strong that I was having to jump out of the bed, and was feeling like I had to jump out of my skin. That hasn't happened in a while now. So, yeah, I think about stuff but I'm not thinking about it like I used to. I can actually sit down not think about what I have to do over here or over there.

When asked whether he'd noticed any changes in his PTSD, pain, depression, or drinking, Mr. H responded,

> Maybe me being more positive. But, no. Not anything that I could really put my hand on . . . except for . . . this is what worked for me. The ability to live . . . the ability to know that I don't have to worry about yesterday or tomorrow, I'll just be living with today and right now. So them things are very big in what I accomplished out of that.

He also said he has gotten a handle on his drinking and now has just one to two drinks a couple of times a week and is no longer using it to cope with pain or negative feelings.

In summary, depression, substance misuse, chronic pain, and functional somatic conditions commonly co-occur with PTSD, and many patients find that they are able to apply mindfulness skills to them as well as to the ways they may be linked. A common thread running through this chapter is that mindfulness practices provide individuals an avenue to shift their way of relating to difficult symptoms or emotions. Throughout the chapter, we discussed how MBIs are thought to help patients manage the inevitable day-to-day fluctuations in stress that can exacerbate both physical and mental health challenges. We also discussed how MBIs afford the opportunity to adopt practical skills to interrupt unhelpful cycles of rumination and catastrophizing, which tend to worsen the clinical course of various psychiatric conditions and chronic pain syndromes. Information was also provided regarding how MBIs can lead to new ways of examining beliefs about the meaning of symptoms, which can lead to improvements in functionality. Although mindfulness practices may not result in a "cure" per se, they can increase patients' sense of agency regarding their symptoms and reduce the level of suffering and distress associated with each condition.

This concludes Part I of this book, which is intended to provide greater knowledge of the landscape of conditions that commonly occur following trauma, along with a description of how increased mindfulness can be of benefit. In Part II, we move on to practical considerations. Chapter 3 discusses important aspects of how to effectively manage and teach individuals in a group setting and Chapter 4 provides practical suggestions for how to teach specific mindfulness practices to people who have sustained trauma.

PART **II** PRACTICAL CONSIDERATIONS

PRACTICAL CONSIDERATIONS FOR OFFERING MINDFULNESS-BASED INTERVENTIONS TO PEOPLE WITH TRAUMA HISTORIES

3

This chapter provides guidance on facilitating mindfulness groups that include individuals with posttraumatic stress disorder (PTSD) and other conditions commonly associated with trauma. Our recommendations are based both on the procedures and approaches we have refined over the past decade offering mindfulness-based interventions (MBIs) to patients in a Department of Veterans Affairs medical center as well as the recommendations of others who have described their approach to offering MBIs to trauma populations in the literature. The suggestions and perspectives provided are intended to be relevant across a variety of settings. Thus, the goal of the chapter is to provide general recommendations regarding the referral process, elements of a pregroup orientation session, inclusion criteria, and issues that are useful to cover in initial group sessions. We then share specific observations about handling group dynamics that may be especially relevant for those with trauma histories. (Note: throughout this and the following chapter, we use the terms *group leader, therapist, facilitator,* and *teacher* interchangeably; likewise, we use *class, session,* and *group* interchangeably.) We conclude with reflections and suggestions intended to highlight practical clinical issues

http://dx.doi.org/10.1037/0000154-004
Mindfulness-Based Interventions for Trauma and Its Consequences, by D. J. Kearney and T. L. Simpson

Referring to Mindfulness Groups

Providers who refer patients to a mindfulness group need to remember that there is no need to convince a patient to enroll. We suggest simply providing a general description of the program along with encouragement to attend an informational session/orientation. The patient can then decide whether the group is a good fit. A brief explanation that learning mindfulness, through techniques such as breathing meditation, helps to reduce stress and manage symptoms seems sufficient as a first step to gauge receptivity and interest before referral. Many patients resonate with the fact that stress worsens overall symptoms for many conditions, which can serve as a useful entry point.

Providers who refer patients with PTSD or other trauma-related issues are encouraged to reassure patients that they will not have to share their trauma story in the group (Magyari, 2015). The referring provider should also ask the patients whether they have concerns about taking part in an MBI class. For example, although we have found that many patients with PTSD are willing to enter a group, some are reluctant to participate in group programs for a variety of reasons. These reasons may include concerns about personal safety, reluctance regarding sharing personal information, a tendency to become irritated or angry and associated worries about personal control, or trepidation about meditation and being silent with their own thoughts and feelings. It can be helpful for the referring provider to assist the patient in airing her or his concerns. Depending on the concerns, it may be appropriate for the referring provider to work with the patient and MBI team to help the patient identify ways to cope constructively should any of her or his concerns about taking part in the MBI be realized. We recommend that such a patient-affirmative approach be taken rather than attempting to provide blanket reassurances that are likely to be unsatisfactory. If the referring provider has an ongoing relationship with the patient, it can be helpful to make a plan to check in regularly to help the patient integrate the new experiences and perspective learned in the MBI. Another consideration for referring therapists is to obtain necessary consents so that the MBI leader can consult with the referring therapist if needed (Magyari, 2015).

Orientation Session

Providing an orientation session for people who either self-refer or who are referred by a provider helps them decide whether the program is a good fit. Requiring attendance at a group or individual orientation session may also commonly encountered when teaching mindfulness in a group format to people who have sustained trauma.

PREGROUP CONSIDERATIONS: GROUP COMPOSITION, ELIGIBILITY, REFERRALS, AND ORIENTATION AND INTAKE PROCEDURES

We have found that carefully consideration of each step of the process involved in forming MBI groups increases the likelihood that the intervention will be successful. Many of the issues described here will necessarily vary according to the clinical context in which the groups are offered.

Group Composition

Our approach has been to offer MBIs as groups composed of individuals with a variety of clinical problems, including PTSD, chronic pain, and depression. In certain contexts it will make sense to offer mindfulness-based intervention (MBI) courses that are geared specifically toward individuals who are struggling with the aftermath of trauma, whether in the form of PTSD or another trauma-related condition. In other settings, MBI courses will be open to all comers, which almost certainly means that some individuals will and others will not be significantly impacted by trauma. Although forming groups composed entirely of individuals with trauma histories may allow tailoring of teaching in ways that are beneficial, a potential benefit of heterogeneous groups is that the shared experience of the group is squarely placed on learning mindfulness rather than attempting to address PTSD symptoms or other trauma sequelae; it may help prevent sidetracking into problem-solving. In our setting we have allowed patients both to be referred by clinicians or to self-enroll if they elect to do so. We have allowed people with PTSD, including complex PTSD, to self-refer and enroll in an MBI as long as they do not meet specific exclusion criteria as recorded in the medical record (see below); we have not found that this is associated with safety concerns or adverse events. However, we recognize that the acceptability of this practice is likely influenced by the setting in which the MBI is provided. We practice in the context of an integrated health care system in which most patients have received some prior education about PTSD, have very chronic PTSD, and are actively engaged in other forms of care. In our setting, we consider the practice of allowing self-referrals as consistent with a patient-centered, patient-driven care model that encourages opportunities for patients to engage in self-care in conjunction with professional care (Krejci, Carter, & Gaudet, 2014). The above comments are intended to provide perspective on the range of practices regarding referral practices and clinical composition of groups, which will vary according to the setting and clinical context.

Eligibility Criteria

When developing eligibility criteria for participation in a general mindfulness group (i.e., a mindfulness group that is not focused on treating a specific diagnosis or condition), we suggest a policy of broad inclusiveness. There is growing evidence that mindfulness interventions provide benefit across multiple conditions, which includes aspects of both physical and mental health. Because people commonly present with a wide range of overlapping physical and mental health concerns, mindfulness programs with broad eligibility criteria are likely to be more attuned to the needs of individuals seeking care. Framing MBIs as a wellness or self-care activity, rather than a mental health treatment, might help some people engage in care, given that some people perceive a stigma associated with mental health treatment (Dutton, 2015). Alternatively, in other contexts, providing MBIs as a form of therapy for specific conditions can be the most effective approach and can allow the visit to be coded as therapy.

For eligibility criteria for a general MBI offering, we suggest accepting all individuals who have a desire to participate in a mindfulness group after attending an orientation session and who do not meet one of the following exclusion criteria: (a) actively psychotic; (b) poorly controlled bipolar disorder with mania; (c) substance use disorder or alcohol use that poses a safety concern or is associated with an inability to keep appointments (though as discussed later in this chapter, mindfulness approaches have been successfully used in the context of substance abuse treatment); (d) suicide attempt or suicidal ideation with intent or plan, self-harm within the past month, or psychiatric hospitalization within past month (unless the group is specifically offered in a setting with appropriate safety monitoring in place for these individuals); and (e) those in the immediate crisis phase following trauma (Magyari, 2015). Although we recognize that learning mindfulness could potentially benefit individuals with some of these exclusion criteria, they are listed because of concerns that some conditions could disrupt the group process or would require closer safety monitoring than is possible in a large group setting.

help to reduce attrition from the group by helping to ensure that people understand what the program entails. We have not conducted individual face-to-face orientation sessions for individuals with PTSD before beginning the course, although individual orientations may help to build trust and have been recommended by others (Dutton, 2015; Magyari, 2015). An orientation session helps to minimize the potential for surprises that could lead to participants dropping out of the group. Ideally, the orientation session should be conducted by the teacher or therapist who will lead the group, which allows prospective participants to establish rapport with the group leader and better determine whether the program is a good fit. The orientation session also provides an opportunity to clarify that, unlike traditional psychotherapies, MBIs do not have symptom reduction as a primary goal. Would-be participants should be informed that symptom reduction may well occur, but the main focus of MBIs is on cultivation of openness to experience through increased capacity to observe one's thoughts and feelings, awareness of reactivity, shifts away from patterns of reactivity, and development of greater capacity for self-compassion and kindness.

The first interface with the MBI team is an important factor in setting the tone and establishing trust for all would-be participants. For patients with prominent trauma histories, these first impressions are especially important, as it is often difficult for them to enter into unfamiliar situations and they may be less inclined to persist if they perceive that things are disorganized or MBI team members lack attunement or understanding.

Intake Procedures

In our setting, we conceive of MBIs as adjunctive courses meant to promote improved self-care and well-being, and thus we do not conduct formal psychosocial intakes. This means that we do not obtain details about patients' trauma histories unless they spontaneously offer them. During the course of an MBI class sequence where the group is often large (typical MBSR classes range from 15 to 25 members), we have found that it is uncommon for individuals to share this information with the group, although such sharing is not actively discouraged. What is encouraged in MBIs is becoming more aware of experience, and sharing trauma-related material may be appropriate if relevant to their present-moment experience (Magyari, 2015). Thus, MBI teachers do not necessarily know which patients in their classes have trauma histories and therefore approach them all as though each one is likely to have endured hardship and as though each one has significant strengths, both realized and untapped.

BUILDING A CONTAINER OF TRUST AND FRAMING EXPECTATIONS: THE FIRST FEW SESSIONS

Establishing a sense of trust is particularly important for trauma survivors. Providing an MBI in a manner that fosters both a feeling of safety and a sense of predictability is likely to enhance the ability of trauma survivors to more fully engage in mindfulness practices that are new to them and are perhaps somewhat challenging.

Guidelines for Participation

When establishing a mindfulness group, it is important that group members feel there is enough openness to allow their voice and other voices to be heard, to feel that it is acceptable to not speak, and to feel that their questions, comments, and observations are held by the group in a way that is supportive and nonjudgmental. There also needs to be enough structure to keep individuals or the group from going off topic or from shifting into a mode of advice-giving. Setting out clear expectations is likely to be helpful for all MBI class participants, but it is especially critical for those who may have difficulties with trust or are apt to feel very anxious in new situations. In this and the following sections, we share examples and approaches that help to establish the group as a container of trust.

In Session 1, it is important to carefully review a set of guidelines for participation; an example is provided in Exhibit 3.1. The purpose of the guidelines is to set expectations for the group and to begin establishing group norms on which participants can rely. Topics covered include attendance, whether sharing is required, confidentiality, and guidance about interacting with other group members.

Rules of Engagement

A shorter, pithier version of the guidelines for participation is expressed in a saying used by one of our mindfulness teachers. As originally described by Parker J. Palmer (2009), the rules of engagement can be distilled as: "No fixing, no saving, no advising, no setting each other straight" (p. 115). It is helpful to review these guidelines in the first session and to emphasize that this means not giving advice. If at times in the mindfulness series a participant begins to advise or give advice to others, it can be helpful to restate these guidelines. This can be a simple "let's make sure not to fix others," or it could include recognition that "the advice seems to be coming from

EXHIBIT 3.1. Guidelines for Participation

1. **Please be on time.** We will cover a lot in our time together, and you may miss something important to you if you are late. On the other hand, if you cannot avoid being late, please be sure to come in quietly anyway. It is better to be late than to miss a session.

2. **Do the homework.** Set aside 30 to 45 minutes each day for your formal practice, even if it means 30 to 45 minutes less sleep. Many people find that 45 minutes of meditation can result in benefits that go beyond those derived from sleep.

3. **Maintain confidentiality.** Keep what is discussed by others in the group absolutely confidential. You are free to discuss your own experience with others outside of class.

4. **Be supportive, but do not try to fix others.** The greatest support for this practice is a respectful, considerate environment. We support one another by simply listening and not offering advice or trying to solve one another's problems. The most transformative learning happens when we each arrive at our own realizations in our own time. We will try to create an environment where each person can begin to see beyond all the "shoulds and should-nots" to what is actually true for him or her in each moment.

5. **Focus on the present moment, not past or future experiences.** Use "I" language to talk about what is going on in your body and mind, and remain present-centered. For instance, "I notice thoughts of leaving class because of the tightness in my chest right now"; "I feel like I can't breathe." We will refrain from storytelling. Instead, consider what you are experiencing *here-and-now*: e.g., "right now, I notice tingling and burning in my legs." The most important aspect of this class is your experience in this moment.

6. **Communicate your concerns.** Please let the teacher know if you are having any difficulties. You may do so in the group or speak privately with the teacher. Time to talk before or after class or on the telephone will be available.

7. **Be respectful of the group process.** If you will be absent or must leave early from a class, please notify the instructor or program coordinator beforehand.

8. **Plan to turn off your cell phone during class.** Since this class is about establishing and sustaining attentional focus, cellphones, texting, and email can be very disruptive, especially during periods of guided mindfulness practices. You are invited to see this class as your own personal time, a kind of miniretreat within your day. Please make sure that you have made any essential calls, texts, or emails before class has begun.

9. **Do not bring visitors.** No one is to bring spouses or friends to any of the classes who has not been enrolled in the class from the beginning.

Note. Data from Santorelli, Meleo-Meyers, and Koerbel (2017).

care and concern" and "each person will benefit from finding his or her own path in his or her own time, so it's best to avoid giving one another advice." For some MBI participants, this will be a very different kind of experience, and it may be difficult for them to refrain from offering advice, particularly if advice-giving functions as a way to avoid discomfort or their repertoire for connecting with others is limited. Gentle persistence on the part of the MBI teacher on this point is important both for maintaining clear boundaries and for instilling the idea that distress does not need to be "fixed" and that it is tolerable.

Mindfulness Training as a Complement to Other Health Care

We suggest framing participation in a mindfulness group as a complement to, rather than a replacement for, usual care. This topic can be covered in both the orientation session and the first class session, and it can include encouragement to discuss with participants' health care providers how learning mindfulness fits with their overall treatment plan. Describing this framework can help patients enter into mindfulness training with more realistic expectations than might be the case if they were coming to the group with either the fear that their primary providers might disengage from them or that mindfulness training will provide a fix for their problems.

It is important to note that what constitutes "usual care" is highly variable across settings; some integrated health care systems have rich resources available to patients (e.g., VA care or some managed care settings), whereas other settings are more limited in terms of the specific additional services available to patients. Moreover, some individuals may choose to participate in a community- or hospital-based MBI as their sole approach to addressing their psychiatric or emotional issues, including PTSD and other trauma-related conditions. Thus, we encourage MBI teachers to have a list of the mental health and substance abuse resources in their communities, particularly those that are low-cost or offered on a sliding scale, to provide in the event that any of their class participants need referrals to formal treatment.

Attending the Group

When discussing attendance, we suggest that if people must be late because of other obligations, they enter the group as quietly and unobtrusively as possible. In addition, we sometimes suggest that when others or they themselves arrive late, it provides an opportunity to bring awareness to one's own reaction patterns. Do they experience judgment? Curiosity? Compassion? What arises? In this way it can be helpful to weave the inevitability of some people arriving late (as well as other disturbances) into the theme of the classes, and to frame these disturbances as opportunities for learning. The overarching framework is to invite participants to think of the class as a laboratory for their minds and bodies. We have found that some individuals with trauma histories find it challenging when others are late, whether because they are startled by the inevitable noise of someone entering the room, irritated by what may be perceived as disrespectful behavior, or feeling unsettled by the unpredictability of such situations. Similarly, for those who come in late, there may be a host of thoughts and feelings to note. Again, we suggest encouraging people to notice what comes up in these situations and to meet whatever arises with curiosity, openness, and compassion for oneself. In this way class participants are encouraged to build the capacity for equanimity in the face of irritating challenges both in class and in their day-to-day lives.

It may also help to explain to participants that when people come and go a lot in the series, it can disrupt the flow of the class and make it difficult for the group to maintain cohesion and a solid container of trust. It can be helpful to point out that showing up can also be considered a form of support and generosity for others.

Encouraging Effort and Accountability

Mindfulness leaders often encourage participants to view the class series as a valuable opportunity to learn about themselves and reshape well-worn habit patterns—and that some effort is required. Mindfulness teachers are encouraged to speak directly from their own experience about the importance of mindfulness practice in their lives and to reflect briefly on how the sustained effort required has gradually helped them to navigate life's difficulties successfully. It can help to remind participates that as they proceed in the course the teacher will be doing the same practices as those taking the class. To convey how practice can be uncomfortable and results can be delayed, some mindfulness teachers use the analogy of going to the gym. For example:

> If we want to gain physical strength, we wouldn't expect that working out would produce this change in 2 or 3 weeks—it would naturally take much longer for us to gain strength. In this way, attending the mindfulness group is like going to the gym. To build any kind of strength or capacity, it will take some time—at least several weeks.

In this example, the teacher advises participants to let go of short-term expectations and commit to at least eight weeks of practice before checking in on their progress.

Also, to promote accountability, when people know they will miss a week, we ask that they mark this beforehand on the attendance sheet as an "informed absence; I.A." We strongly encourage participants to attend the first class, which lays the groundwork for the series, and advise people who must miss classes (especially the first two) to consider passing on this series and signing up at another time.

The above examples are provided as ways of promoting accountability and effort in mindfulness groups. We suggest that teachers find their own way of expressing the importance of effort and commitment as appropriate for the population they are working with.

Balancing Class Expectations With Acceptance
That People Are Doing Their Best

Along with encouraging people to be on time and to set aside time each day for practice, teachers should encourage each person to simply "do the best they can." So, while teachers need to acknowledge that a certain amount of discipline is needed in the class structure, it is important to model an attitude of kindness and nonjudgment. Participants should be encouraged to do their best, but to not beat themselves up if they cannot fulfill all the expectations of the class. Maintaining such a dialectic can be especially important for people who have either held themselves to unattainable standards or have let themselves off the proverbial hook too easily, both which are common responses to challenge among individuals with prominent trauma histories.

Advising Participants That Learning Mindfulness
May Initially Increase Their Stress

Some people enter a mindfulness class with the expectation that their stress levels will promptly decline. In fact, this often does not occur. As a person becomes more aware of thoughts, feelings, and body sensations, the experience is sometimes that of increased stress. Rather than explaining this possibility to people, we suggest weaving it into group discussions if comments by group participants suggest an increase in stress levels. We like to quote Kabat-Zinn (2005) from *Full Catastrophe Living*: "It can be stressful to take the Stress Reduction program" (p. 2). Framing the experience in this way can help participants readjust their expectations and prepare them for the challenges and opportunities ahead.

It can be particularly helpful for those with PTSD to hear that such an increase in stress or symptoms is normal and not an indication that something is wrong or that they are doing the practices incorrectly. When such issues arise, it can be an opportunity to invite participants to notice what is coming up, to be curious, and to view it as a valuable opportunity to learn new ways of relating to difficulty, rather than perhaps settling quickly on a definitive interpretation of what it might mean. The mindfulness teacher can guide inquiry into the experience through gentle, concrete questions such as "What is happening right now in your body? or What are your feelings? Can you be with them in a friendly way?" (Magyari, 2015, p. 147). These remind participants that sometimes when we are quiet and there is time and space for thoughts and feelings that have been avoided, consciously or unconsciously, it can be unsettling and hard and that this is okay. In the next chapter we provide additional concrete examples of ways of working with specific mindfulness practices (i.e., sitting meditation, walking and other movement meditation, compassion or loving-kindness meditation) in the context of PTSD and trauma histories.

Explicitly Describing the Approach Taken in a Mindfulness Group and Contrasting It to Other Support- or Process-Oriented Groups

At the outset, it can help to acknowledge that the format of many groups is to discuss and process what has happened up to this point in group members' lives, and that *while this is often valuable, it is not the purpose of this group*. Instead, the format of mindfulness group discussions is to learn about, discuss, and practice mindfulness, which involves becoming more aware of present-moment experiences. To make the point more strongly, some instructors clearly state that "this is not group psychotherapy, nor a support group (though people are generally supportive of one another)—it is a mental training, and everyone is training together." This may come as a surprise and possibly a relief to some people. It can help establish a "container" where participants understand that while they may hear some of the other's stories, they do not have to take them on. Additionally, for those with PTSD and other trauma-related conditions, setting these parameters can help provide reassurance that they do not need to share their trauma history.

Reading

When discussing homework, if a book or other reading materials are provided as part of a mindfulness series, we recommend framing reading materials as supplemental and optional, whereas doing the meditation practices is the primary homework. Although we acknowledge that reading about mindfulness is often helpful, for many people the amount of time available for activities outside of class is very limited. Describing reading materials as an additional resource they can delve into after the program ends helps to make the point that the primary learning is experiential (i.e., the learning occurs through mindfulness practices).

THE GROUP FORMAT

Many people with trauma histories have trepidation about participating in groups, as doing so necessarily entails coming into contact with numerous other individuals, many if not all of whom are unknown. For those whose traumas involved other people, contact with unknown others can be especially stressful and challenging. We find it helpful for group instructors to remember that many of their new class participants are likely feeling very much outside their comfort zones; as instructors work with those participants, they should build a group context that the individual members will eventually find supportive and useful.

Opportunities for Growth

Although the group format can present numerous challenges, it also affords opportunities for growth. Many people find that the group provides motivation and support to practice, both inside and outside the classroom. For example, the group often fosters a sense of accountability for homework practice, despite obstacles. Sharing in the group can also be therapeutic for many people, especially in the presence of individuals who are similarly dealing with physical and/or emotional pain. Another way we encourage participants to utilize the opportunity of the group format is by inviting them to engage in the practice of active listening as a form of mindfulness meditation. Instructors may prompt participants to notice what comes up for them as they listen to other group members. Ask participants to question themselves periodically regarding whether they are really listening or are perhaps in their own thoughts, what they are feeling about what is being said, and what thoughts and emotions are coming up for them.

Such questions can help participants observe their reactions to others as learning opportunities, thereby capitalizing on the unique challenges of working in a group and turning them into opportunities for growth. For instance, rather than becoming lost in judgments about others, or pushing away feelings of annoyance or irritation, participants should be encouraged to turn their awareness to these internal experiences as events worthy of interest and understanding. It may also be useful to ask participants to note if they experience similar reactions to people when they are outside of class. If so, why not use the experience in the mindfulness group as an opportunity to work with these reaction patterns? The teacher facilitates this process by modeling interest and curiosity about these reaction patterns. For example, "How great it is that you are noticing that annoyance is coming up for you. Are you able to stay with this and be curious about it?" If the teacher models this during interactions with one or two participants, it often serves as an example that is useful to others in the group.

Managing the Group and Facilitating Participation

Often participants in mindfulness groups appreciate the chance to share their experiences about the practices and learn from one another's perspectives. However, many are bothered when group members share if it steers the conversation to issues they consider off-topic or inappropriate for a mindfulness group. Holding the group accountable is encouraged, and providing clear structure is helpful in this regard (Martinez et al., 2015). At the beginning of class, it helps to tell the group that there may be times when the instructor will need to interrupt the conversation. For example, if people are "in their story," the instructor might invite them to become more present with their bodies and what they are experiencing in the moment. Or, because of time constraints and an effort to adhere to the curriculum, the instructor might need to stop a conversation and move on. Saying this at the outset helps mitigate hurt feelings later. Additionally, the instructor needs to have techniques at hand to cut people off in a dignified manner, to politely redirect, and use skillful inquiry. Simple phrases of bringing people back, if they become tangential, might include interjections or questions from the instructor such as, "Can you bring it back to the exercise we're discussing?" "I need to ask you to come back to the topic at hand," or "I need to ask you to pause." Don't be afraid to be direct. We have heard repeatedly from participants that they appreciate directness and clarity from the instructor.

For some people, sharing in a group can be an anxiety-provoking experience. This anxiety often subsides over the course of the group for many, but for others it remains a challenge, motivating them to stay very quiet even though they may be experiencing difficulties or may have observations they would be inclined to share under other circumstances. We suggest inviting participants who do not share frequently to try to share more. Instructors can invite people who are not comfortable speaking to notice this tendency and consider getting out of their comfort zone. It can be helpful to provide the reminder that this would occur within the safety of this group.

Given that in most groups there are those who like to speak and those who do not, one way of encouraging participation by all group members is to suggest that they use group discussions as an opportunity to practice mindfulness—if they are the kind of people who like to talk, they might be encouraged to watch that need and see what it feels like to hold back. What do they notice? Conversely, with people who do not easily speak in groups, it may help to frame this as an opportunity to practice taking risks and to take their place. These encouragements should be extended as a gentle invitation; the option of remaining silent should also be acknowledged.

This practice often creates a greater sense of safety for those initially reticent to share.

Attending to Everyone in the Room

A challenge for the group leader is to stay tuned in not only to the person sharing but also to others in the room who are taking it in. At times, other group members may experience painful emotions or memories while one shares a difficult story or experience. This may be because the experiences resonate and remind some of similar situations from their own lives. This is often a time to encourage participants to stay with their own experience, to touch into the felt sense of the body, and to be curious about why the discussion has brought up specific emotions within them. In the present moment, are there memories of the past? What thoughts are here now? What emotions arise? Can these experiences be held in a greater field of awareness, with kindness, curiosity, and compassion? Is it possible to stay with this experience, grounded in the breath and the body? In this way, the instructor can help other group members to grow in understanding as they listen to the experiences of others. Encouraging these ways of working with challenging group material can be helpful for group members with and without trauma histories, but they are especially important for those with PTSD, as they run counter to habitual avoidance and dysregulated emotional responses to such triggers.

PRACTICAL CONSIDERATIONS

Depending on the clinical context in which an MBI is being offered, there may be opportunities to offer classes to particular groups of individuals, and there may be capacity to have more than one instructor lead a group. In this section, we share some observations about offering women-only groups in particular, as well as potential benefits to having two instructors if staffing permits.

Group Composition

Some female participants prefer a women-only mindfulness group because they feel uncomfortable in a room with men, especially if they have experienced sexual trauma. Participation in a mindfulness group invites vulnerability, and while some discomfort is natural and encouraged, there is a point at which it is too difficult to practice. However, many women do not have an issue participating in a group with men, and participating in a mixed-gender group could serve as a step toward dealing with avoidance patterns toward men. In support of this is evidence indicating that women with PTSD who participate in mixed-gender groups do as well or better than men in terms of PTSD symptom reduction (Felleman et al., 2016). We suggest that mixed-gender mindfulness groups for women with histories of interpersonal trauma should be offered to women if they are open to it and feel prepared to take this step. However, it is not necessary for patients to confront their most difficult sources of stress at the outset. When mixed-gender groups are offered, make it clear in the orientation process that there will be both men and women in the group. In this way, women can make an informed decision about whether they are ready to participate in a mindfulness group with men. If possible, women-only groups should also be an option available for women with PTSD.

Facilitators

Typically, a single instructor appears to be sufficient for mindfulness classes. However, when working with large groups (e.g., 15–25 participants), a second instructor can be helpful to check in on individual participants, particularly during movement practices. Also, for many people, hearing mindfulness instructions from instructors with different personalities, teaching styles, and gender can be beneficial. An added benefit is that a second instructor can effectively teach by modeling mindful listening and attentiveness as the other instructor speaks.

Although some individuals may prefer a female instructor, many appear to have no preference. Some women with histories of interpersonal trauma could likely benefit from opportunities to approach their discomfort, fear, anxiety, or anger in a women-only format, and in this situation a female instructor is preferred. In other settings, there may also be benefits to having male instructors, as they can provide helpful modeling of mindful self-reflection and emotionality. Many men have been taught to show limited emotion or to believe that emotional communication makes them appear weak. The presence of a male instructor who consistently demonstrates that one can be strong yet mindful and emotional can provide powerful corrective lenses for both male and female group participants. Male instructors who effectively balance the head and heart and communicate this synergy with clear, accessible language will be most effective.

In general, the most effective means of connecting with the group is to keep the emphasis on learning mindfulness as the shared experience.

We have found that teachers who embody sincerity, humility, authenticity, and direct experiential knowledge of mindfulness practices are readily accepted by the group. It is very helpful for teachers to have an ongoing personal mindfulness practice and when teaching to speak directly from (and not beyond) their own understanding. If the instructor sometimes shares his or her personal struggles with learning mindfulness, it can solidify the bond with the group through the common shared experience of learning mindfulness. One of the most powerful ways of learning mindfulness can be through interacting with a teacher who embodies a mindful way of being. If the teacher naturally embodies warmth, openheartedness, curiosity, humor, and acceptance, it can help to bridge the gap between divergent life experiences and foster a strong sense of trust and connection with the teacher (Ahlin & Kjellgren, 2016). We discuss teacher qualifications and characteristics in more detail in Chapter 5.

CHALLENGES FACED BY PEOPLE WITH PTSD WHEN LEARNING MINDFULNESS

One of the primary goals of this book is to help mindfulness teachers who work with trauma survivors gain a working knowledge of the clinical manifestations of PTSD, as well as how mindfulness can be applied to some of the mechanisms thought to maintain the disorder. We do not, however, suggest that mindfulness teachers attempt to frame class discussions around PTSD symptoms, use the clinical language of PTSD symptomatology, or attempt to focus on symptom reduction. Rather, we suggest keeping the focus on learning mindfulness. When experiences are shared that may be related to PTSD, such as hypervigilance or emotional or behavioral avoidance, we suggest using everyday language to work with these experiences (e.g., by noticing thoughts, feelings, and bodily sensations). In fact, in our experience working with individuals with PTSD, the term "PTSD" is almost never used by instructors.

Opting In

Understanding that PTSD symptoms include avoidance, which can make participation (or sharing) in a group challenging, can help instructors better facilitate group discussions. Understanding that there may be many possible reasons for reluctance to participate can also be helpful. Potential issues could include anxiety about being judged by others, concern about not being able to control one's anger responses, or feeling that one's experiences or perspectives are so extreme as to not be understandable by others. Encouragement to share, while acknowledging that being open in this way may go against deeply ingrained tendencies, can sometimes help people to engage. An invitation to share can be made while still offering the option to opt out if needed (along with encouragement to practice opting out without judgment). Framing participation (or showing up to class) as an act of courageousness can also be helpful.

Working With Feelings

For some individuals with PTSD, emotional numbing may occur as a consequence of longstanding PTSD. Indeed, alexithymia, or the inability to recognize and label feeling states, is common among those with PTSD (Frewen, Dozois, Neufeld, & Lanius, 2012), so instructors may find it useful to select specific, basic feeling and emotion terminology (e.g., "Moving your attention to your lower back, you might notice what feelings or emotions arise for you. Are there feelings of sadness or anxiety? Or maybe relief or contentment? Whatever feelings are there, notice them and return your attention to your lower back") both when guiding meditation practices and when facilitating class discussions. It can also be useful to matter-of-factly state that emotional numbing can occur following trauma along with a discussion of how mindfulness leads to an enhanced ability to experience emotion. This can help class participants understand the rationale for the practice, which in turn can serve as a motivating factor for continued practice. Encouraging patients to experiment with the naming and noting of feelings can be a useful tool. Instructors should also recognize that prevalent emotions among individuals with PTSD may include pervasive feelings of shame and guilt. When these emotions are experienced, individuals are encouraged to hold these feelings with kindness and self-compassion, which in turn is reflected by the instructor.

Noticing Reactions

Hypervigilance and exaggerated reactivity may also be evident at times in mindfulness classes. For example, as related by one instructor, when a behavioral emergency was called out over the hospital public address system, many patients were triggered. During class, the instructor guided the participants to notice the experience in their minds and bodies with mindful awareness. In this way it was used as a learning experience. Some individuals also find it uncomfortable when sitting with their back toward the door or when others walk behind them. Some report keeping their guard up and feeling uncomfortable opening up to strangers. Instructors may give suggestions on how to work with these feelings: for instance, by noticing them come and go, along with urges to react to them (e.g., the urge to leave the class).

In helping group members work with all of the aforementioned challenges they face and others, we have found that it can be useful to make explicit connections regarding how mindfulness training can be used to address common unhelpful thought patterns. Many class participants seem to appreciate assistance by the instructor in making the link between rumination, depression, and mindfulness. The concept of rumination is typically introduced early in the class series and is addressed throughout the course series, often by naturally inserting comments during group discussions. Briefly sharing findings from the scientific literature, which report a marked reduction in depressive relapse after learning mindfulness, can help to reinforce the value of the practice. Suggestions can be given to notice the problem-solving tendency inherent in rumination and contrast this "doing mode" with the "being mode" fostered by mindfulness practice. Providing concrete examples during meditation practice throughout the course series helps group participants practice recognizing when they are slipping into old patterns and gives them alternatives to bring to bear. Infusing the examples with reminders to let go of judgment and to bring self-compassion to the fore can also help patients begin practicing kindness toward themselves and to repair the tendency to engage in negative or harsh self-talk.

As described in Chapter 2, patients with PTSD often have one or more additional mental health conditions or physical health concerns. The material provided in that chapter can help mindfulness instructors have a better sense of the challenges often faced by their group members. Chapter 2 provides a theoretical rationale as well as practical guidance for teaching mindfulness to people with depression, chronic pain, somatic conditions, and substance misuse. In the remainder of this chapter, we provide additional practical suggestions pertaining to the process of teaching mindfulness to individuals with PTSD.

Notes on Safety and Well-Being

Patients with suicidality require close monitoring to ensure safety. If this is not possible, as noted earlier, we recommend excluding patients with suicidal ideation with intent. Inclusion of patients with active suicidal ideation may be appropriate and feasible when groups are led by mental health clinicians and each patient is engaged in another form of mental health care. There is evidence that this approach is safe and beneficial to patients with suicidal ideations who participate in MBSR (Serpa, Taylor, & Tillisch, 2014).

Should an instructor recognize that a participant appears to be depressed or very anxious, the instructor may check in with her or him after class. The instructor may urge that person to make contact with his or her other providers for additional support. Early in the class series, as well as in the orientation session, patients should be encouraged to utilize their existing resources (e.g., therapists, other groups, friends, family) for support in processing issues that may arise. As noted earlier, instructors not operating within a health care system should have familiarity with available mental health and substance abuse resources in their community, including websites and phone numbers for suicide and crisis lines, should they need to provide referrals for additional treatment or support.

Working Productively With Addictions

As described in Chapter 2, it is safe to assume that some class participants will have issues with alcohol or drugs and may use these substances to facilitate avoidance, to "feel normal," or to feel anything. While it is not necessary or helpful to refer frequently to alcohol and drugs or to addiction, periodically bringing awareness of addiction dynamics to formal meditation instructions and into discussions of applying mindfulness skills in one's daily life can help class participants better recognize when and how they can employ what they are learning to mental and behavioral processes that often operate on autopilot. For example, during class discussions of the value of learning to stay with discomfort, the instructor can ask people to reflect on strategies they use to avoid discomfort, which could include alcohol or drugs. Doing so can help tie what otherwise might be disparate, abstract ideas together so they are more useful and can help destigmatize problems with alcohol and drugs so that those for whom this is relevant can approach these issues with more self-compassion and less shame.

Chronic Pain and Expectations

In working with chronic pain and mindfulness, instructors need to manage expectations about the realities of pain reduction. Sometimes people will come to an MBI because they heard it could "get rid of their pain." These are often the people who end up being the most disappointed. Emphasize that it is not about the pain per se but about one's relationship to it. The conceptual model and evidence base for MBIs in relation to chronic pain are discussed in Chapter 2, and specific suggestions for working with pain during meditation are provided in Chapter 4.

SUMMARY

In this chapter, we discussed specific practical considerations that should be taken into account when forming and leading groups composed of individuals who have sustained trauma. We described suggested practices for educating referring providers and applying exclusion criteria, and we discussed a number of issues that often arise involving group dynamics. We also reviewed suggested rules of engagement and creating a container of trust, which are of issues of great importance if a teacher or therapist is to effectively manage groups that include trauma survivors. We turn now to Chapter 4, in which we provide reflections and suggestions for teaching specific mindfulness meditation practices to individuals with prominent trauma-related issues.

4

REFLECTIONS ON TEACHING SPECIFIC MINDFULNESS PRACTICES

In this chapter, we provide a brief discussion of practical considerations in teaching mindfulness that are common across various practices followed by suggestions for teaching specific mindfulness practices, including body scan meditation, sitting meditation (or breathing meditation), mindful movement (yoga and qi gong), walking meditation, and loving-kindness meditation (LKM). Of note, teaching trauma-sensitive mindfulness primarily involves adhering to good teaching practices for mindfulness rather than significantly altering how the practices are taught—an observation that has also been made by others with experience teaching MBIs to people with trauma (Magyari, 2015). Some of the elements of good teaching practices include taking care to build a container of trust (described in Chapter 3), having the understanding and ability to respond appropriately to challenges experienced by participants, maintaining appropriate boundaries, and providing clear instructions.

The skillful and effective use of language by the teacher or therapist is particularly important, and teachers and therapists should strive for a balance between encouraging kindness, steadfast effort, courageousness in

http://dx.doi.org/10.1037/0000154-005
Mindfulness-Based Interventions for Trauma and Its Consequences, by D. J. Kearney and T. L. Simpson

the face of difficulty, and a willingness to accept limitations. One general suggestion is to use language in the form of an invitation as a way of promoting empowerment and choice on the part of the patient; for example: "I invite you to bring your attention to the feeling of the breath in the body." Allow patients to go at their own pace, through phrases such as "When you feel ready, allow your eyes to open, then make your way back to the circle."

We suggest interspersing brief psychoeducational information over the first several sessions of mindfulness-based interventions (MBIs) to help participants understand how psychological approaches such as MBIs can help them cope with stress, symptoms of conditions like posttraumatic stress disorder (PTSD), depression, and substance use disorders, as well as chronic physical pain. Although MBIs emphasize experiential learning, and most teachers encourage participants to see for themselves what may or may not be helpful to them in these practices, it can be reassuring to patients to learn about how clinical studies suggest a benefit of MBIs for these conditions. The need for psychoeducation is based on qualitative research we have performed with veterans with a variety of trauma-related sequelae (Martinez et al., 2015), as well as the understanding that for most people it is counterintuitive to intentionally allow oneself to feel pain, whether physical or emotional, rather than finding ways to distract oneself from it or attempt to fix it. Providing a framework with psychoeducational materials can help facilitate greater trust and openness to exploring a different path.

The need to provide some understanding of the purposes of the practices was described by two participants in qualitative interviews we conducted at our site. One participant reported,

> It's hard for me. I think it's more because I'm not understanding the whole concept of it. . . . Sometimes it's like I can't understand why they're doing it and why I'm going to scan, what the purpose is really and how it's going to help me. Sometimes I get lost in that and I'm not able to focus on anything else. I'm not able to move on.

Another participant described this as

> I didn't like doing the body scans 'cause it brought attention to my pain. . . . And I spend more of my time trying not to focus on my pain. And it was like, "Okay, you're asking me to focus on my pain, and that makes no sense to me." . . . We're supposed to resist the pain, that's what we're taught: resist the pain, not to approach and accept it.

When one discusses the fact that meditation practices can be challenging, it can be helpful to mention our natural and understandable tendency to avoid pain or discomfort, and to acknowledge that when remedies to alleviate discomfort are available, it can sometimes make good sense to pursue them. The concept is then introduced that when we reflect on it, we see that despite our best efforts, emotional and physical pain often cannot be made to go away, and no day is without discomfort, difficulty, or dissatisfaction. Participants can be invited to reflect further about how persistent efforts to avoid pain or discomfort can gradually limit our lives, which can be particularly pronounced in PTSD, as it is characterized, in part, by avoidance. Depending on the group context, it may also be useful to point out that some efforts to avoid pain or discomfort, such as over-use of alcohol or drugs and staying excessively busy, can lead to even more pain and distress. That may contribute to an unproductive cycle characterized by short-term distraction coupled with lower thresholds for handling pain and discomfort effectively, as well as increased health and functional consequences.

When the concept of the inevitability of some degree of discomfort is introduced, it is also useful to highlight the value of learning new ways of working with discomfort, which from the perspective of MBIs involves becoming more curious and interested in the experience of emotional and physical pain, including our reactions to it. This process of examining our experience more closely can be succinctly described as a process of moving toward difficulty rather than avoiding it—one in which it helps to proceed with gentleness and kindness. When describing this approach, we sometimes introduce the expression "If it is in the way, it is the way." Many people seem able to relate to the concept that moving toward a difficult situation with an eye toward skillfully navigating obstacles in our path holds value. Potentially beneficial outcomes can be described as including increased awareness of what is going on with one's emotions and body, which can form the basis for more informed choices about how to respond to stressful situations, how to pace oneself, how to be gentler with oneself, and how to perhaps be less reactive or angry in the face of emotional and/or physical pain or trauma reminders.

One of the cornerstones of teaching mindfulness is working with judgment, which inevitably arises in the course of all of the meditation practices whether in the form of self-criticism over one's perceived inability to do them properly or more generally in the form of noting preferences for this or that aspect of the experience (e.g., "If the teacher doesn't make that person stop talking, I'm not coming back," "Everyone else seems to be doing fine, but I can't sit still at all," "Why do they allow it to be so hot in here?"). Encouragement to notice these tendencies of our minds is at the heart of mindfulness training. Judgment also frequently comes up around the various practices, and here too, we encourage participants to adopt an attitude of kindness and curiosity when aversions or preferences for specific practices arise (e.g., "I don't like the body scan," or "The body scan doesn't work for me because I always fall asleep," or "I really love the breathing meditation"). It is important for the instructor to support all the practices so that participants continue to challenge their learning edges. Participants are encouraged to view each practice as an opportunity to learn more about themselves, including how they deal with situations that are uncomfortable or that do not meet with their preferences. What is it about a specific practice that they find difficult? If there are ideas that they cannot do this, are those ideas true? Can they experiment with approaching each practice with openness and a beginner's mind, knowing that no two practice sessions are the same?

Another opportunity for working with judgment often arises naturally because many mindfulness courses are offered in hospital or clinic settings that are not always quiet and calm. There may be overhead announcements or loud conversations in the hallway outside. Often the noises and activity are intermittent, which can startle participants who are attempting to focus on their breath. Oftentimes reactions to such interruptions can be reflexive and strongly negative. Although it is generally a good idea to attempt to minimize distractions by not holding mindfulness classes in or near busy areas, unplanned interruptions seem to occur with regularity, which provides participants an opportunity to examine how they respond. Inviting participants to notice their initial responses to loud noises and voices and to meet those responses with kindness and curiosity can help them recognize that while they may not be able to choose their immediate reactions, they do have choices about whether they fuel frustration and anger or whether they consciously choose to return to their breath.

We also find it helpful to frame participants' decision to undertake an MBI course and to stick with the practices as an act of courage. Expressing gratitude for their presence and honoring their willingness to be with themselves as honestly and directly as they are can often provide helpful encouragement for those who find the practices challenging. One instructor sometimes tells the group that when she looks out across a room of people in silence and stillness, she thinks it is one of the most courageous things each one could possibly be doing. Participants may be encouraged by hearing about their teachers' own early meditation experience—if they hated sitting still, how hard it was, how they just wanted the leader to ring the bell, how they struggled with self-criticism—and what kept drawing them back to the practice. It can be helpful to acknowledge that it is so much easier to get up and seek pleasure or avoidance and that it takes real courage to just stay, stay, stay.

Similarly, we often remind participants that in the context of meditation, practice does not make perfect. As we note repeatedly throughout this chapter, and indeed throughout this book, the idea to convey is that minds always have a tendency to wander; we will likely frequently feel squirmy and unable to get physically comfortable when we meditate; and we will have judgments about ourselves, one another, and the practices. All of this is normal and provides opportunity for further inquiry and deepening of self-compassion. Essentially, there are no boxes to check off or milestones to achieve.

THE BODY SCAN

The body scan is a central component of many meditation courses. It typically involves a slow, guided invitation to bring attention to each part of the body and to notice the sensations that arise. We have not shortened or otherwise altered the format of the body scan for people with a history of trauma, and this has not been associated with excessive distress in our experience. Offering the body scan in this way, without significant modification for individuals with PTSD, is consistent with other reports of clinical acceptability in the literature (L. L. Davis et al., 2018; Kearney, McDermott, Malte, Martinez, & Simpson, 2012, 2013; Kimbrough et al., 2010; Polusny et al., 2015). That said, many individuals, and particularly those with trauma histories, may find the body scan challenging. Thus, for a person with PTSD, it is particularly important to ensure that the class space is of sufficient size that people do not feel crowded and that it feels private and safe (e.g., there are not frequent interruptions or anyone not in the class using the space), which helps patients to engage in the body scan as well as the other mindfulness practices.

We suggest providing instructions that balance steadfast effort with kindness and acceptance of limitations, particularly when working with individuals who have sustained trauma. The option should be left open for people with PTSD or chronic pain to shorten the body scan if they do not feel they can participate otherwise; this can be included as part of general instructions. Thus, we encourage MBI teachers to have patients engage in the practice in ways that feel accessible to them. For some, this will mean that they practice, at least initially, with their eyes open, while others, because of physical limitations, will choose to sit in chairs, lie prone with their knees bent or supported by a bolster, or use the an "astronaut pose" with calves up on the seat of a chair. Others may position themselves away from the group if space allows. A matter-of-fact and flexible approach that encourages patients to find where and how to practice the body scan will acknowledge that it may be difficult for some without implying fragility or weakness or leading some patients to feel they have to ask permission to alter the practice to make it doable for them.

When participants have difficulty practicing the body scan, we advise explaining that even practicing for a few minutes can be better than not doing it at all, and it can be built upon each day. Moreover, we have found that most people with PTSD are able to practice for the full duration of the exercise without reports of excessive distress, but including the above permissions for modifications is beneficial to some people. Ultimately, helping participants feel empowered to engage in the practices in ways that are doable for them is more likely to benefit them than attempting to adhere to a standard protocol.

The practice of bringing attention to each body area is usually coordinated with the breath, such that participants are encouraged to systematically breath into and sense each body region. This practice develops the ability to direct and sustain attention and fosters an experiential shift to the being mode of mind. The shift into a felt sense of beingness involves feeling into experience with an attitude of openness and allowing, without attempting to change, judge, or fix anything. Further description of the being mode of mind as compared to the doing mode of mind is provided in Chapter 2. While sensing each part of the body, a person is also encouraged to notice the thoughts and emotions that arise and to allow these to pass in the background. Many people find that staying present in one's body is challenging either because they are carried away by thoughts of the future or memories of the past or because the sensations or feelings in the body are painful or uncomfortable. As a result, people sometimes have either positive or negative reactions to body scan exercises. Awareness of these potential, often unspoken, responses can be helpful when leading the practice.

It helps to maintain a warm, neutral tone as each new body region is introduced and to move at a pace that is not too slow; steady verbal instructions can help to rein in a wandering mind. When participants are working through the body scan, it can also be useful to periodically encourage them to notice sensations that are often easier to feel, such as the feeling of body against the floor or chair, or movement of the belly or torso with breathing. During the body scan, the leader asks participants to notice what sensations are present, such as how relaxed or tense muscles feel, or whether there is tingling, coolness, warmth, fullness, or numbness, and reminds participants to approach their experience with an attitude of curiosity, openness, and kindness. During the practice, practitioners are also asked to check in with themselves about any thoughts, feelings, or general reactions to specific body parts. It can also be helpful to acknowledge and normalize the possibility that a person's experience in the body scan might involve feeling emotionally or physically numb, or they might experience feelings of distress. Providing examples of nonjudgmental ways of working with thoughts and feelings, particularly around body parts or regions that are painful or that are associated with traumatic memories can help participants shift their relationships to their bodies. For example, an MBI teacher trying to help trauma survivors who find the pelvic region challenging might say,

> If you find yourself tensing or maybe having a harder time staying present as you settle your attention on your pelvis, it can be helpful to remember to breathe into this region of your body just as you would any other and to bring yourself back if you find your mind wandering. If this is painful for you or if it brings up fear or anger, for example, notice and acknowledge these feelings and return to the experience of your breath in your body.

Because physical pain is so common for individuals who have experienced trauma and because individuals with significant physical pain can find it difficult to engage in mindfulness practices that encourage stillness and present-centered focus, we offer a number of ideas for addressing pain in the context of the body scan and later when leading sitting mindfulness meditations. For example, one might encourage class participants to work with pain in the following way:

> As you bring your attention to your lower back, you might notice some tension or pain. If this is the case for you, you might see what it's like to direct your breath into this painful area and to feel some tenderness for this part of yourself. If focusing on this area of your body brings up painful memories, notice this and acknowledge it. Breathe into this area, aerate it, and notice from moment to moment whether the sensations change. Just stay with the experience noticing whatever arises with an attitude of curiosity and kindness. Also notice any thoughts or emotions in the background. If you find yourself feeling angry or sad that you are hurting, attempt to greet it with kindness. And now after the next exhale let's move the focus up a bit to just between your shoulder blades.

This is an example of bringing mindful attention to pain in a specific body area and helping patients stay with it for a few moments in the face of challenging feelings or memories that might come up for them, then letting go and shifting attention to the next body area during the course of body scan practice. The patients can thus learn to separate thoughts and beliefs that arise as part of the pain experience from the sensation of pain itself, and in the process they may find that beliefs they held no longer seem to be true. In our experience, most patients with significant physical and emotional pain find it possible to practice in this way.

For some people with severe physical or emotional pain centered in a specific part of the body, it is too difficult to move on to the next body area given that their attention is strongly drawn to the painful area. If this is the case, we suggest patients remain with the painful sensations—continuing to breathe into the area, bringing an attitude of kindness and curiosity to the experience, and noticing as the sensations change slightly from breath to breath. It can also be helpful to suggest noticing thoughts that arise during the experience, and to specifically mention the possibility of catastrophic thoughts such as "I can't do this" or "if I focus there, it'll remind of being raped and I'll lose it" or judging thoughts such as "focusing on my pain is stupid." Encouraging them to hold these ideas with curiosity, noting that they may or may not be true, can be helpful. The instructor may then offer that if they feel ready, they can attempt to let go of this area and continue with the body scan practice, perhaps with the painful area in the background but shifting the main focus of attention to the area covered in the body scan. Alternately, if it feels necessary and more helpful to remain focused on the painful area for the duration of practice, that is also fine. In working specifically with physical pain, we invite participants to observe the sensation of pain and their physical, cognitive, and emotional reactions *to* pain. What is happening to their breathing? Are their muscles tense or relaxed? What story do they tell themselves *about* the sensation? Encourage them to observe the story without identifying with the story. Emotions can be observed without being swept away by the emotion. Ask them to discover for themselves how some cognitions and emotions escalate pain while others deescalate it. For group members with significant trauma histories, it can be helpful to acknowledge that sometimes the stories we tell ourselves about our pain can be very painful in and of themselves and might even feel overwhelming and yet they can be approached with the same openness and kindness as any other thought or feeling one might experience.

SITTING MEDITATION (OR BREATHING MEDITATION)

Sitting or breathing meditation is a cornerstone of mindfulness practice. It can help create space for learning more about oneself, one's thoughts and feelings, and ways one habitually processes or appraises situations. Breathing meditation is intended to develop an enhanced ability to direct and sustain attention. The object of attention—in this case, the sensation of the breath—is for most people a neutral sensation that is neither pleasant nor unpleasant, which, along with its constant presence, makes it an accessible object of meditation. Also, the sensation of the breath is inherently subtle and closely associated with sensations of the body and emotions. Cultivating the ability to stay with the breath provides an avenue to develop increased awareness of emotional and physical states, including subtle emotions and their relationships with physical experiences. Essentially, breathing meditation can provide foundational groundwork for learning how to slow down and interrupt established habit patterns in one's thinking and responding. Over time and with mindfulness practice, when people are caught up in cycles of thought or difficult emotional states, they become increasingly adept at shifting attention to their breath and to sustain that attention while allowing thoughts and emotions to pass in the background. The act of disengaging or letting go of cycles of thoughts and emotion, and shifting attention to the breath, creates "space" and allows thoughts and emotions to be regarded with curiosity and openness.

In an exit interview at our site, one participant described how the teacher helped him to learn breathing meditation:

> He told us to put one hand over our heart and one hand over our belly, and the one over our belly was to help us know we were getting breath into our belly and that would reaffirm what we were doing. And like I said the first time we did the mats, after about ten minutes, I was able to breathe deeply enough that I was able to do that.

Many course participants carry this teaching on past their formal involvement in the mindfulness course, adopting a regular practice of sitting or breathing meditation that becomes part of their daily routine. Indeed, research suggests that more than 80% of mindfulness-based stress reduction (MBSR) participants use breathing meditation as a coping technique over the course of long-term follow-up (Kabat-Zinn et al., 1986). Such ongoing practice is helpful in coping with pain and stress, and participants often report that the breathing meditation helps them step out of reaction patterns and allows them to exercise sounder judgment and greater self-control. One participant with PTSD summarized how to use the breath to interrupt reaction patterns:

> The biggest thing is when I see something is building up inside of me, as far as, like I feel like I'm going to get angry, or get upset, I check in with myself. So I would stop, and then I say, "okay you [got to] take a deep breath," and I would. When I breathe, I don't just breathe in and hold it, I do an eight count up and then an eight count back out. (Schure et al., 2018)

Learning how to change their response to a situation by breathing, rather than reacting in a habitual fashion, appears helpful for those with PTSD. A qualitative study of 15 individuals with PTSD who took part in

MBSR found that breathing through stress emerged as a consistent theme (Schure et al., 2018). Indeed, for many people with PTSD it becomes a regular part of their daily routine to handle stress and negative emotions. Another MBI participant from our site described the influence of breathing on reaction patterns:

> When I find myself . . . when I'm walking along or driving along, and I find I'm not breathing, at that point I am so tense and so stressed, that a deep breath brings me back or slows me down . . . and I need to get control. . . . I understand now that my breathing is part of the process of me getting control or taking control back. So, it's directly connected to how I see myself handling a particular situation or how I'm engaged. I know when I . . . can get so engaged that I will stop breathing, and that's when anger and irritation comes on.

Another summarized the utility of breathing meditation:

> I'm able to deal with it a whole lot better using my mind or using breathing to help control a bad situation. Normally I would just fly off the handle, say anything, but stopping, taking time to breathe, and do a little thinking, I can resolve getting into an argument over whatever was said, so I just deal with it differently instead of just jumping right off chewing your head off.

When an instructor teaches sitting meditation, it is useful to keep in mind that this practice can be challenging for a host of reasons. For some it can seem an anathema to simply sit and do nothing, while for others the prospect of sitting still can lead to claustrophobic feelings of entrapment or greater agitation and restlessness. For some people, sitting still and being quiet with oneself can feel scary in that it runs counter to habits of staying busy and distracted from painful thoughts and feelings. Indeed, some participants find sitting meditation to be more difficult than the movement practices. One participant described his challenge with breathing meditation as

> I don't think I would have any challenges at all doing the practices if I could breathe like a normal person. And we're working on that through my primary care physician. That's the problem with meditation, you have to be able to deep breathe.

If group members do not speak about these challenges openly, instructors can provide reassurance by lightly touching on some of these possibilities during the first few class sessions. Hearing that these sorts of experiences and judgments are common experiences others have dealt with can help participants see that their responses are not aberrant and are workable. It is also important to matter-of-factly set a positive frame for staying with the sitting practice as a means of building the "mindfulness muscle" by strengthening one's ability to be with what is uncomfortable or unpleasant in a less reactive way. We find it helpful to acknowledge that sitting practice can be difficult, to remind participants that it is intended to serve a useful purpose, and to provide kind encouragement for continued practice. We often encourage participants to adopt a courageous attitude of moving into difficulty and to bring an attitude of strength and kindness to this endeavor.

In addition to the challenges of sitting quietly with oneself, many, if not most, beginning meditators find that sitting still quickly becomes physically uncomfortable or even painful. We find it helpful to ask participants to notice the tendency to want to move or shift to minimize pain in meditation practice and to suggest that if they need to move or shift during practice in response to pain that they do so with full awareness. Participants are asked to turn toward the pain, to investigate with openness and curiosity the actual sensations, and to stay with the sensation "as best we can in that moment." In this way they are asked to be open to the moment-to-moment sensations of pain or discomfort. This requires kindness and self-compassion. An emphasis in the instructions on kindness, as well as permission to "just do your best" can be a helpful way of conveying the need for kindheartedness when approaching pain. It is often helpful to ask participants to breath into the area of pain or to "aerate" the pain, which helps them to with and investigate the moment-to-moment experience of the body. Another potentially beneficial approach can be to ask participants if they see the pain as solid and fixed and therefore stuck and firm, like a board. If they experience pain in this way, they can be asked to breathe into and through the area of painful sensations. It can be helpful in this process to imagine it as more porous—more like a sponge than a rock. This slight shift in perception can be very helpful to some people.

However, as with all the practices, it is beneficial to include in the general instructions encouragement for participants to trust their intrinsic wisdom. This is important for all participants and can be especially helpful to people with significant trauma histories, as learning to trust oneself and take care of oneself accordingly can be beneficial both within the context of the MBI class and potentially in other parts of their lives. Thus, we explicitly remind participants that if they feel it is necessary for them to disengage or adopt a different form of practice, it is perfectly acceptable. We endeavor to interlace such reminders with comments on how important it is to balance accommodating discomfort with the knowledge that it is often necessary to lean into difficulty if one is to grow. In addition, this can be a useful opportunity for the mindfulness teacher to provide instruction about working with judgment. This can take the form of asking participants to notice whether judgment arises, either as a comparison to others in the room or to an internalized standard. If that is the case, we invite participants to view it as an opportunity to work with this aspect of experience—to notice judgment—and then to continue practicing with kindness and steadfastness as best they can.

In keeping with the need to provide a flexible atmosphere in which group participants may make adaptations to practices to accommodate their needs, if participants have significant physical limitations, sitting in chairs rather than sitting on a cushion on the floor is preferred. When needed, participants are free to adapt the seated posture further, with the addition of cushions, or to practice breathing meditation while recumbent, to accommodate pain or disability. One participant described his need to find a suitable posture as

> I have a hard time doing the seated meditation, but if I can cross my legs on a cushion my posture is much better, it's a better meditation. The seated ones, the injuries hurt sitting. That's probably one of the things that hurts the most. But it doesn't hurt in a cross-legged position.

With regard to meditating with one's eyes open or closed, either method is perfectly acceptable, which is important for some individuals with PTSD to hear, as they may experience anxiety sitting in a room with relative strangers with their eyes closed. Some instructors will mention that if a person prefers to meditate with eyes open, it is perfectly acceptable, and that in fact some meditation traditions teach this form of practice. Despite this invitation to practice with eyes open if needed, we find that nearly all participants with PTSD choose to practice meditation with eyes closed. When providing guidance for meditating with one's eyes open, it is helpful to suggest that participants choose a neutral spot a few feet in front of them down low so that they have a restful visual posture and others in the group do not feel they are being stared at. Dutton, Bermudez, Matás, Majid, and Myers (2013) successfully adapted MBSR to included eyes open meditation for low-income women with PTSD and histories of intimate partner violence on the basis of focus groups and individual interviews.

MINDFUL MOVEMENT

Some MBI class participants are surprised to learn that there are mindful movement options, since their understanding of meditative practices often involves images of serene-appearing people sitting very still. For more active or restless people, the introduction of mindful movement practices can be quite welcome, indeed. Others, however, may find it challenging to pay close attention to how their bodies feel when moving, or they may feel self-conscious if some of the practices are difficult or feel awkward. Instructors are encouraged to be patient and gentle when introducing the various mindful movement practices, and to present them as equally valuable alternatives to forms of meditation practiced in stillness. Mindful movement can also provide a valuable opportunity to ask participants to notice any habits of self-judgment as well as the tendency to strive for mastery or perfection.

Yoga and Qi Gong

Many participants enjoy yoga and qi gong. Mindful movement practices seem to be particularly helpful for pain relief, and with appropriate modifications mindful movement practices, including yoga and qi gong, are not too difficult for most individuals with physical limitations and those who have perhaps been reluctant to focus on their bodies because they were the site of painful trauma experiences. Importantly, although in other settings it may be appropriate for a yoga instructor to touch participants (after obtaining permission) to help adjust their posture, in the setting of teaching MBIs to trauma survivors we recommend that teachers or therapists not touch participants.

Of note, when MBSR is taught, significantly simplifying the yoga sequence proposed in the original MBSR curriculum allows those with physical limitations to participate more fully and successfully. Such simplified yoga sequences and qi gong practices appear to be accessible and acceptable to those dealing with chronic pain and trauma-related mental health symptoms. Engaging in moving meditation also appears to serve the purpose of demonstrating for some participants that they are capable of more movement than they previously thought and that they are able both to gently push their bodies and to fully inhabit them. One participant we interviewed described this as

> I have had a lot of back problems . . . you know throughout the years your back gets beat up. And, when I wake up in the morning, it's even difficult to just sit up in bed. If I do the yoga practice and I do it on a daily basis, generally an hour or so after I get up. . . . It takes away a lot of that tension and it makes the day a whole lot easier to move around. Not only is it physically invigorating but is also very mentally invigorating. The better I feel physically, the better I feel mentally. I don't' feel fatigued, beat up . . . that kind of thing. So, the yoga practices have been wonderful.

These can be empowering realizations, with positive short- and long-term consequences. Chair yoga, which uses a chair as a prop and support, is also a viable option for many individuals. Here is how one MBSR participant described modifying the yoga postures so they work for him:

> I try to do the yoga part of it and the different stretches and that. I don't cross my feet, I don't cross my legs, I kind of just sit there. I do it kind of differently to accommodate me.

When giving participants options and modifications for doing yoga, it is suggested that they also be given the option to opt out. It can be supportive to gently urge participants to give it their best effort or perhaps to participate in only small movements (e.g., raising and lowering arms) if they have significant physical limitations.

It can also help for the group leader to point out that body sensations always occur in the present moment, and that awareness of these sensations can help to anchor us in the here and now. In movement practices, whether by stretching or walking, we often elicit physical sensations in the body, which can help to draw our attention to experience in the present moment. The instructor can reflect that although thoughts of past and future also occur in the present, their focus is on other than what is occurring now, and that focusing on the past and future tends to limit our awareness of what is going on in our lives in the present—which is when our lives are lived. In this way, the concept that physical sensations can be used as an anchor to ground us in the present moment is introduced.

Walking Meditation

MBI course participants often find that walking meditation provides them with the opportunity to slow down and be in the moment while doing something simple, repetitive, and familiar. Repeated experience with such slowing down can facilitate a shift in perspective and encourage a way of engaging in being mode rather than doing mode in the midst of activity. For this reason, many participants incorporate walking meditation into everyday activities. For some, walking meditation can be initially uncomfortable or mystifying, but many find that they come to appreciate the practice more over time. Those with physical disabilities and balance problems may find walking meditation too challenging and quite possibly unsafe, so we recommend they substitute sitting meditation as a more viable option. From a logistical perspective, walking meditation requires rooms of ample size or nearby hallways or outdoor spaces where participants may still be in visual contact with the instructor and the rest of the class.

In describing his reaction to walking meditation, a veteran who participated in an MBSR course had this to say:

> Typically we are going from point A to point B on a constant basis, and the walking meditation gave us the opportunity to slow down to be in the moment, to not have an end goal to reach. That was a different aspect for me. I'm used to going from here to there and getting things done; whereas being in that moment and just taking time to focus on the steps, the movement, your breathing, was very different. That stands out to me.

One of the unique aspects of practicing walking meditation in the context of a mindfulness class is that it can involve 15 to 20 people moving about in a room together. Thus, there is a need to balance maintaining a quiet focus on one's own experience while simultaneously navigating around and accommodating others so everyone can move safely about the space. It can also offer an opportunity for participants to observe their habitual responses. "Do I have a tendency to feel anxious and irritable if others are in close physical proximity?" "When there is an opportunity to yield or keep going do I tend to respond one way or the other?" "How am I feeling about there being movement behind me that I can't see?" "What sort of thoughts and feelings arise when my back is to the door or when access to the door is blocked by others?" "Am I able to stay in the felt sense of my body despite these challenges?" MBI teachers can pose such questions aloud at the beginning of a walking meditation or raise one or two during the debriefing discussion afterward to both provide participants with examples of ways they might work with walking meditation and to normalize the sort of thoughts that are likely going through their minds.

This handful of example questions reflects ways walking meditation can provide very direct practice for mindfully navigating one's life outside of class. Inviting participants to notice without judgment what arises for them as they work with their breath, notice their bodies in space, and navigate around and with the others in the room can start cultivating the seeds of mindfulness on the fly and the ability to pause and regroup in the midst of everyday life, as the following quote from an MBSR participant illustrates:

> [When] you're actually doing it, you start to realize that meditation is not something you necessarily do when sitting down or laying down. It can be just a part of your life, you know, a way of being. . . . I think walking meditation is kind of an intro to the realization that you can have that presence, that presence when you're doing the body scan, you can have that all the time when you're talking to people, when you're moving through the world.

LOVING-KINDNESS MEDITATION

LKM is a practice that is designed to repeatedly elicit feelings of kindness and goodwill toward oneself, feelings that are hypothesized to counteract shame, guilt, and self- and other alienation. Additionally, the cultivation of positive emotions through LKM may be helpful for those who have difficulty feeling positive emotions, such as love and affection, and could help repair the numbing and constrictive symptoms that so frequently are part of the emotional landscape for individuals with PTSD. In LKM practice, participants sit quietly and call to mind their intention (i.e., what they hope or wish) for self and others, working through various categories of persons (e.g., a good friend, a benefactor, a difficult person, oneself) and sequentially invoking positive intentions for them that may include safety, happiness, health, and ease. Notably, in the Buddhist record, LKM was taught as an antidote to the strong emotion of fear (Salzberg, 1995), which is a dominant emotional experience in PTSD (Foa & Riggs, 1993), and so it is not surprising that for many it appears to be a more accessible practice when distress is high than meditation practices focused on following the breath.

LKM is often introduced in MBSR courses during a Saturday all-day retreat and is offered as an additional tool in one's toolbox. Thus, it is useful to advise participants that some practices may be more helpful in certain life circumstances, or during certain periods of life, and for this reason we introduce distinct but interrelated practices. For example, it can help to have familiarity and facility with both sitting meditation and mindful movement practice (e.g., yoga, qi gong, walking meditation), and it can also be helpful to have some experience and understanding of LKM as one navigates life's difficulties. In addition, there is growing interest in developing and evaluating entire MBI courses focused on LKM (Kearney, Malte, et al., 2013; Kearney et al., 2014) and other methods of cultivating increased self-compassion (Neff & Germer, 2013).

The phrase *loving-kindness* derives from the Pali word *metta* (or *maitri* in Sanskrit), which can be translated as "love," "unconditional friendliness," or "loving-kindness" (Salzberg, 1995; Thera, 1994). Whether MBI teachers plan to simply briefly introduce LKM or focus an entire course around the practice, it is helpful to be clear that the words *loving-kindness* are intended to describe an emotional state that is not a sentimental love or a feeling of passion. Rather, it can be described as an unconditional friendliness, benevolence, and openness toward experience—even difficult experience. Classically, four phrases are used, such as "May you be safe," "May you be happy," "May you be healthy," and "May your life unfold with ease." Gradually and systematically, LKM phrases are extended to other individuals or categories of people, including oneself, a benefactor, neutral persons, those who have caused difficulty or harm, and all beings, changing the phrases as needed (e.g., "May you be safe" becomes "May I be safe"; Salzberg, 1995).

While practicing LKM, it is helpful for instructors to suggest that participants notice and feel any positive emotions that arise after repeating the phrases of positive intention and to notice if there is a sense of reluctance, hesitation, or aversion for oneself or others. A person practicing LKM is encouraged to notice the experience—regardless of whether it is love or a feeling of deficiency or aversion—with a nonjudging, kind, and open attitude. Also, during LKM, when a person becomes distracted by thoughts that arise, reminders to notice the distraction and to return to the phrases without judgment are helpful supports for the practice. While practicing LKM, a person is also encouraged to remain grounded in the feeling of the breath and the body. Walking meditation may also be adapted for LKM practice; the rhythmic nature of walking is typically synchronized with the repetition of LKM phrases. Outside of class, informal LKM practices are encouraged as well; participants are asked to practice LKM toward themselves or others during everyday activities such as walking, eating, washing the dishes, or standing in line at the grocery store.

The repetition of LKM phrases can be conceptualized as creating a safe holding environment for distressing thoughts and feelings. The repetition of phrases of positive intention is intended to bring to the surface positive emotions that may be difficult for some people to access, including those with trauma-related conditions such as PTSD. By eliciting feelings of warmth and kindness, loving-kindness practices are intended to build a person's capacity to acknowledge and tolerate, rather than avoid or suppress, distressing thoughts, images, and feelings. In LKM, this holding environment is facilitated by self-directed phrases of positive intention, which enhances the ability to feel, rather than avoid, painful emotional states. Buddhist teacher Jack Kornfield succinctly described this process of experiencing compassion in response to pain as "the heart's response to sorrow" (Kornfield, 1993, p. 93). Similarly, an MBSR participant said that "loving kindness brings in the love, hard core. . . . When you do loving kindness, you're working directly with light. You're consciously bringing love into the situation."

In our experience, LKM elicits a range of reactions among those who have experienced trauma. Some find it challenging and uncomfortable, while others find it essential in their process of healing and describe it as having a positive impact on themselves, their family relationships, and their ability to interact with strangers. For some, it helps them feel greater kindness and love toward themselves as well as others.

Because LKM can elicit a mix of strong reactions, it is important to emphasize that not only is it not a problem that difficult thoughts and feelings often arise during LKM practice, but it is an expected and therapeutically desirable part of the process, including, and perhaps especially, for those with trauma histories. As with other forms of meditation, when practicing LKM through repetition of the phrases, participants are invited to notice whatever thoughts, emotions, and feelings arise. This might include limiting beliefs; painful emotions (e.g., shame, guilt, anger); or feelings of inadequacy, isolation, hesitation, or aversion to self or others. Again, consistent with other types of meditation practice, in LKM the practice is to greet these experiences with kindness, to notice them with curiosity and without judgment, then eventually to return to the LKM phrases and the breath without self-criticism. One of the most important pieces of scaffolding that instructors can provide when teaching LKM is to include a comment along the lines of "if while practicing you don't necessarily notice positive emotions, that is fine—you are not doing the practice wrong. In LKM practice, we encourage you to just do it and then to notice whatever arises with an attitude of kindness and friendliness."

In our experience, bringing awareness to limiting beliefs is a very common part of the clinical encounter when teaching LKM to groups of people with PTSD. For example, people often share that they do not think they are deserving of love, or that they are not capable of feeling love for themselves. Or, when asked to call to mind someone who has shown goodwill or kindness to them at some point in their lives, they may respond that they do not believe that there are others who have genuinely acted in a spirit of goodwill toward them. For many, seeing clearly the beliefs they hold surrounding kindness for oneself and others is a new, and often profound, experience. In situations where participants are unable to identify someone living or known who has shown them positive regard, it can be helpful for instructors to help them get creative and perhaps think of a pet who was dear to them or a fictional character who they think would be kind to them. Even if such concerns are not specifically raised by anyone in the group, we find it useful to anticipate that someone in the room is worrying about this and to go ahead and suggest a host of alternative beings for them to focus their practice on.

Another common experience is that the practice of LKM can bring forth a more general feeling of discomfort. Sometimes people do not directly speak to limiting beliefs, such as believing one is not deserving of love or capable of feeling love, but rather they may talk about not feeling comfortable as illustrated by this participant's comment:

> I felt odd in doing it. . . . It's just a practice of something that we don't normally do for ourselves, so I was kind of uncomfortable telling myself that I'm okay with where I'm at in this stage of myself, my being or my situation. That's kind of what was uncomfortable to me.

For many, the act of directing kindness toward themselves can feel selfish, and people sometimes share that it runs counter to the values they were taught in their family.

When beliefs and feelings of discomfort arise during LKM practice, we suggest framing it as a valuable opportunity to bring awareness to these beliefs and feelings, to fully allow the feeling and regard beliefs with kindness, openness, and curiosity. This process is aided by modeling by the instructor and further assisted by normalization of these experiences by the group process. We also find that it is important to note for participants that LKM is not intended to remove painful thoughts or feelings. Rather than attempting to rid oneself of these experiences, it is anticipated that individuals with PTSD and other trauma-related conditions can learn through LKM that pain can coexist with positive feelings because, after all, it is part of being human to experience both. This may help address the phenomenon that we have frequently observed clinically wherein individuals with trauma-histories are afraid to experience positive emotions because it is painful when they end. By relearning (or learning for the first time) that it is safe to feel good and that it is normal to have good feelings (and painful ones) that wax and wane, the often profound emotional numbing typically associated with PTSD may be mitigated (Litz & Gray, 2002).

When teaching LKM, instructors need to have a solid appreciation that the process of choosing LKM phrases involves an element of inquiry and an opportunity for values clarification. Instructors are strongly encouraged to work with various LKM phrases in their own personal practice both to provide themselves with familiarity with this particular form of meditation and to have firsthand experience with the process of coming to one's own set of phrases. As noted above, LKM involves the repetition of phrases of positive intention, and classically four phrases are used: "May I be free from danger. May I have mental happiness. May I have physical happiness. May I have ease of well-being" (Salzberg, 1995). Over time, a person is asked to choose his or her own phrases and to be guided in this choice by reflecting on what is most significant to him or her. It can be helpful to pose a question such as "What is your innermost heart's desire for yourself and others?"

Often people find as they practice LKM week after week that phrases that previously felt meaningful no longer adequately express their wish for self or others. For example, after practicing with the phrase "may my life unfold with ease" for a few weeks, one person with PTSD reflected that this felt passive to him—it reminded him of his habit of avoiding distress or difficulty. What he really wanted was to be more active and engaged. After some discussion with the instructor, he chose the phrase "may my actions be skillful and kind" as his fourth LKM phrase. In this way, clarification of values and one's intentions occurs. The following is a list of phrases used by individuals with PTSD during LKM class sessions:

- May I be safe.
- May I live in safety.
- May I be free from danger.
- May I love and accept myself just as I am.
- May I be free from suffering and the causes of suffering.
- May I be happy.
- May I be peaceful.
- May I be joyful.
- May I be courageous and joyful.
- May I trust in the present moment.
- May I be healthy.
- May I be well.
- May I have mental happiness.
- May I be free from distress and the causes of distress.
- May I be free from fear.
- May I be free and not burdened by past events or fears of the future.
- May I live with ease.
- May my life unfold with ease.
- May I have ease of well-being.
- May I awaken to my wholeness.
- May my actions be skillful and kind.
- May I be wise and skillful.

In the course of teaching LKM, we hear questions about what it is and is not: In particular, we find it useful to be clear that although LKM may lead to forgiveness, it is not the goal of the practice. Also, LKM is distinct from positive affirmations, which tend to be stated as though they are definite personal qualities and are intended to strengthen self-confidence (e.g., "I *am* a good, kind person"), whereas LKM phrases are usually stated as invitations or requests that are intended to tap into the intention for kindness and compassion for oneself and for others (e.g., "*may* I be safe from harm," "*may* you be happy and healthy"). LKM is presented as a practice of intention that cultivates compassion for one's own and others' suffering.

An important method of conveying the shared human experience of suffering (i.e., common humanity) appears to be learning in a group setting. Hearing firsthand the struggles, imperfections, confusion, and sorrow of others often helps to foster greater understanding and compassion. Likewise, sharing one's own struggles, imperfections, confusion, and sorrow with a group of others is often experienced as validating and nourishing. A welcome outcome of expanded understanding that all humans suffer and all desire happiness, which is fostered by LKM, may lead to forgiveness of oneself and of others, but is not the goal of the practice.

In sharing our observations about teaching specific mindfulness practices to trauma survivors, we have sought to provide practical advice and commentary that will enable mindfulness instructors to bring to each class session a gentle, steadfast confidence in the practices, oneself, and the class participants. In this chapter, we discussed the importance, when one teaches to people who have sustained trauma, of the skillful use of language, creating a container of trust, respecting boundaries, and responding to challenges faced by participants, which includes offering options for adapting practices as needed to help with engagement. These aspects of teaching MBIs to trauma survivors can also be considered teaching in a manner that reflects best practices for mindfulness more generally.

In Chapter 5, we discuss another important aspect of teaching effectively: the experience, training, and personal characteristics of the teacher or therapist. A teacher who naturally models a mindful way of being, especially in challenging situations, can provide very impactful teaching through her or his words and actions. When there is palpable distress in the room, the ability of the teacher to greet the experience with friendliness, interest, and nonreactivity is an important component of teaching MBIs. We discuss teacher or therapist qualifications and characteristics in the next chapter, along with suggestions and reflections for sustaining the practice of teaching over time.

5

MOVING FORWARD

In this book, we have described how mindfulness has the potential to reshape the ways in which trauma survivors relate to experiences in the here and now. Mindfulness has been presented as potentially helpful across a range of conditions commonly borne by trauma survivors, including posttraumatic stress disorder (PTSD), depression, chronic pain, and substance use disorders. But can mindfulness really be applied as a generic intervention across a range of conditions? Other researchers have cautioned against assuming that mindfulness will necessarily result in benefit for multiple disorders unless the factors maintaining the disorders in question are addressed (Teasdale, Segal, & Williams, 2003). In this view, neglecting the need to understand how mindfulness can address factors known to maintain specific conditions "is likely to lead to enfeebled and misplaced applications of mindfulness training" (Teasdale et al., 2003, p. 157). In other words, it may be very important for mindfulness teachers and therapists to understand the mechanisms at play in psychiatric conditions if they are to effectively help patients with these problems. For example, highlighting key mechanisms of depressive relapse

http://dx.doi.org/10.1037/0000154-006
Mindfulness-Based Interventions for Trauma and Its Consequences, by D. J. Kearney and T. L. Simpson

and educating clients about the framework for understanding why relapse of depression occurs have been shown to result in improved outcomes for people with recurrent depression who participate in mindfulness-based cognitive therapy (MBCT; Piet & Hougaard, 2011). As another example, educating clients about mechanisms by which mindfulness may deautomatize addictive behavior has been shown to result in improved outcomes for substance use disorders (Garland & Howard, 2018).

It is for this reason that we wrote this book. We think that it will likely help patient outcomes if the mindfulness-based intervention (MBI) group leader understands key mechanisms of disorders and how mindfulness can remediate these factors. Throughout the book we have attempted to explain and highlight mechanisms that maintain or exacerbate conditions that commonly occur among trauma survivors. In our experience, it is possible for instructors or therapists leading general mindfulness groups to learn about these factors and highlight how mindfulness can address these clinically salient features in their class sessions. Educating participants in groups can occur both through including psychoeducational materials and, perhaps more importantly, by responding to situations in the moment as these issues are brought to the surface by patients. By understanding how mindfulness practice can help reshape mechanisms that maintain or worsen conditions that cause immense suffering, we think that therapists and teachers can increase their ability to help patients who are grappling with multiple conditions simultaneously.

An alternative clinical approach would be to sequentially or separately provide interventions to address each condition (e.g., to first address substance misuse before moving on to working with PTSD, chronic pain, or depression). However, in our experience many patients who present with PTSD and related conditions have limited ability to navigate the complexities and logistics of obtaining care in this way, and importantly, often feel that their issues are interconnected and best addressed together in a unified fashion rather than piecemeal (Back et al., 2014). Also, although a greater "dose" of teaching mindfulness specifically for a given condition (e.g., 8 weeks with a greater focus on chronic pain management or prevention of depressive relapse) might result in greater clinical improvement, many patients do not have access to more targeted mindfulness courses. We developed this book in response to the reality that most patients bring multiple needs simultaneously, which is particularly true for trauma survivors, and that MBI group leaders and participants would benefit from understanding mechanisms involved in these conditions. Also, as described in Chapters 1 and 2, many of the facets of mindfulness learned in MBIs that mitigate mechanisms that maintain specific conditions (e.g., rumination, catastrophizing, holding fixed beliefs, the general tendency to persist in the doing mode) appear to maintain or exacerbate multiple conditions. In theory, once these mechanisms are recognized and an appreciation of the role mindfulness plays is gained, the ability to disengage from such habits can be applied across multiple conditions and situations by patients.

Although it requires flexibility and some additional education on the part of the instructor or therapist, the goal is to weave in mindfulness teaching that applies to each of these common conditions over the course of the class series. In our experience, this happens quite naturally, given that patients bring a variety of concerns to the fore during class discussions and during question and answer sessions. As previously mentioned, we also think it is helpful to include psychoeducational materials in the participant workbooks or as class handouts to provide a framework for understanding how mindfulness is thought to influence each condition. But what is likely to be most important is the ability of instructors to respond during class sessions with understanding and appreciation of how mindfulness relates to the conditions being shared.

QUALITIES OF EFFECTIVE MBI TEACHERS

In addition to having facility with both the curriculum and how mindfulness can be applied to mechanisms that maintain specific clinical disorders, the style of delivery is likely to be as important as the content delivered (Teasdale et al., 2003). The style of delivery reflects the understanding of the group leader, and for this reason we think it is important that MBI group leaders have a personal practice of mindfulness. When a person has an ongoing mindfulness practice, the experience among participants is that the teacher or therapist is a co-participant in the group, albeit one who is perhaps a few more steps along the path of learning mindfulness, has experience with the practices, and is competent in his or her role as group leader. In our view, teaching from one's personal understanding—and not beyond it—is fundamental to the process of effectively teaching mindfulness.

This is perhaps particularly important when working with people with trauma and PTSD, where the ability of the instructor to outwardly maintain a stance of nonreactivity, even when significant distress is shared in the group, can serve to model a mindful way of being. The ability of an instructor or therapist to naturally greet sorrow, distress, or painful memories shared in the group with confidence, kindness, and openness can serve as a powerful method of teaching the shift in way of being that group members are being pointed toward. The group leader is, in effect, teaching by example. The natural expression of the instructor or therapist's mindful approach to interacting might outwardly appear to group members as greeting even difficult experience with matter-of-fact acknowledgement, simultaneous with conveying kindness and genuine curiosity about what is being shared, which can help participants to both allow and feel experience, and not react to it. These descriptions are provided in an attempt to illustrate the expanded repertoire of responses available to an MBI leader who has personal experience with the practice; such responses are likely to be less integrated into the responses of instructors without such experience. For these reasons a personal practice appears essential if a teacher or therapist is to naturally model a mindful way of being, which is likely one of the most effective methods of teaching MBIs.

How much training a person needs to teach MBIs generally, and to people with trauma and specifically, is an important and incompletely answered question. Likewise, beyond the process of undergoing training, it is important to consider other characteristics of a teacher and prior experience with meditation that are associated with teaching mindfulness effectively. Various MBIs, such as mindfulness-based stress reduction (MBSR) and MBCT, have developed teacher training guidelines and requirements, which entail attending training seminars, having personal experience with the practices, going to retreats, and being under clinical supervision (Crane, Kuyken, Hastings, Rothwell, & Williams, 2010). Researchers have also developed a measure that attempts to create a reliable, valid metric of teacher competency for MBCT and MBSR (Crane et al., 2012; Crane et al., 2013). From a research perspective, ensuring intervention integrity, including assessing the competence of the teacher or therapist, is an important aspect of high-quality clinical trials.

Another view is that the characteristics of a good teacher are largely independent of a fixed set of requirements for MBI teacher education. This view was expressed in a qualitative study that involved semistructured interviews with 12 experienced mindfulness teachers in which they were queried about important attributes of effective teachers. Themes associated with being a qualified mindfulness teacher included having sufficient compassion and insight, being able to practice and embody mindfulness himself or herself, being open and flexible to changing conditions in the moment, sharing experiences from his or her own life, having a way of being that conveys concern for the well-being of the student, and recognizing the potential in each situation rather than adhering to a fixed curriculum. Also, the teacher should have an understanding of the context in which the teaching occurs (Ahlin & Kjellgren, 2016).

We think that undergoing structured training to deliver a specific MBI and having a personal, and preferably long-standing, practice of mindfulness are both important when teaching MBIs to trauma survivors. The group leader should be able to model for participants a mindful way of being, as described above. Clinically, it is also important that teachers or therapists have facility with the skills and framework relevant to the clinical conditions they will likely encounter so that they can adequately highlight the application of mindfulness to address factors that maintain the disorder (Teasdale et al., 2003).

ONGOING SUPPORT FOR BOTH THE PARTICIPANTS AND THE GROUP LEADER

We now turn to the topic of how to facilitate ongoing support for mindfulness practitioners. This is a critically important issue because the benefits of mindfulness meditation are much like watering seeds that have been planted—seeds will sprout and grow roots if they are watered and the soil is tended; this will allow them to blossom and bear fruit in the future. In the same way mindfulness practice must be nurtured in one's day-to-day life if it is to be helpful in times of stress or challenge in the future. When a MBI course concludes, it is common practice for the teacher or therapist to discuss how participants can engage support to help them continue to develop an understanding of meditation practices. Although occasionally we have met patients who took a MBI course years ago and then— without further support—continued to practice each day with only the aid of a guided meditation compact disc, we think that such unwavering effort without a community of support is almost certainly the exception. Many people express the need for additional structure, ongoing teaching, and opportunities to connect with others who are grappling with similar challenges, to help them deepen and integrate their understanding. For people who complete a MBI course, support could take the form of offering periodic refresher or alumni MBI courses, encouraging participants to form their own sitting groups, or describing the availability of retreats and ongoing classes elsewhere in the community. Each of these options can prove invaluable to people as they strive to continue to practice and integrate their understanding. For many (or, arguably, all?) people, continued support is essential.

Included among those who need support are teachers and therapists who lead MBIs. Although leading groups can in and of itself provide a form of support and nourishment *for the teacher or therapist,* many MBI group leaders practice in settings where other forms of support for teaching mindfulness seem needed. Some MBI teachers or therapists might lead groups in relative isolation from peers with whom they can talk through questions or challenges, whether those challenges involve how to best help people work with distressing emotions or how to navigate the complexities of recruitment, referrals, room reservations, and billing. Although many find support for learning more about the practices through ongoing affiliation with Buddhist groups and by attending periodic Buddhist retreats, those formats may not provide support for addressing more clinically oriented issues, and obviously are not positioned to attempt to address logistical hurdles. Indeed, during our time working with MBI teachers, a frequently expressed desire is for increased availability of avenues to connect with others who teach the practices.

Perhaps one reason why MBI group leaders would benefit from support is that many MBI teachers and therapists may have initially sought out mindfulness practice as a way of healing their own wounds or navigating personal challenges and difficulties. And although mindfulness practice, as well as other steps, may have helped, additional challenges remain, as they do for all humans. Providing routes for connection and mutual support for MBI leaders could foster continued growth in face of personal difficulties and challenges that despite long-standing mindfulness practices, often persist. As described by Jack Engler (2006),

> There's no way to practice meditation or any spiritual path that is immune from the anxieties, needs, belief structures, emotional patterns, or dynamics of our own personal history and our own character. At the end of the day, we still have to work with sides of ourselves we perhaps hoped spiritual practice would make unnecessary. (p. 19)

We suggest that MBI teachers and therapists take steps to regularly engage a community of peers, which might take the form of joining (or creating) local organizations of MBI teachers, attending regular retreats or sitting groups for MBI teachers, or regularly gathering in informal social settings for support and connection. Although we do not offer more concrete solutions for MBI leaders in terms of support, we hope that highlighting this issue might serve as a useful reminder that leaders of MBIs often need support along the path as well.

CONCLUDING REMARKS

Over the course of this book we have highlighted what at this point remains a partially tested possibility—that offering MBIs in the clinical setting to those who have sustained trauma can lead to positive change and growth. As described in each section of this book, there are plausible mechanisms that can be understood not only by mindfulness group leaders but also by patients seeking help for these chronic conditions. Although more work needs to be done, through the concerted efforts of multiple individuals we are beginning to glimpse the many ways that mindfulness meditation can help people live more fulfilling lives in the face of often daunting circumstances. It is our hope that the information and ideas conveyed in this book focused on teaching mindfulness meditation to people who are suffering in the aftermath of trauma will in turn influence the work of others, so that treatments and approaches aimed at helping those who have sustained trauma can be can be further refined.

References

Addante, R., Naliboff, B., Shih, W., Presson, A. P., Tillisch, K., Mayer, E. A., & Chang, L. (2018). Predictors of health-related quality of life in irritable bowel syndrome patients compared with healthy individuals. *Journal of Clinical Gastroenterology.* Advance online publication. http://dx.doi.org/10.1097/MCG.0000000000000978

Afari, N., Ahumada, S. M., Wright, L. J., Mostoufi, S., Golnari, G., Reis, V., & Cuneo, J. G. (2014). Psychological trauma and functional somatic syndromes: A systematic review and meta-analysis. *Psychosomatic Medicine, 76,* 2–11. http://dx.doi.org/10.1097/PSY.0000000000000010

Ahlin, K., & Kjellgren, A. J. (2016). Prerequisites for teaching mindfulness and meditation: Experienced teachers from different traditions share their insights. *Journal of Yoga & Physical Therapy, 6,* 243. http://dx.doi.org/10.4172/2157-7595.1000243

Allen, M., Bromley, A., Kuyken, W., & Sonnenberg, S. J. (2009). Participants' experiences of mindfulness-based cognitive therapy: "It changed me in just about every way possible." *Behavioural and Cognitive Psychotherapy, 37,* 413–430. http://dx.doi.org/10.1017/S135246580999004X

American Psychiatric Association. (2013). Trauma- and stressor-related disorders. In *Diagnostic and statistical manual of mental disorders* (5th ed.). Washington, DC: Author. http://dx.doi.org/10.1176/appi.books.9780890425596.dsm07

Amutio, A., Franco, C., Pérez-Fuentes, M. C., Gázquez, J. J., & Mercader, I. (2015). Mindfulness training for reducing anger, anxiety, and depression in fibromyalgia patients. *Frontiers in Psychology, 5,* 1572. http://dx.doi.org/10.3389/fpsyg.2014.01572

Amutio, A., Franco, C., Sánchez-Sánchez, L. C., Pérez-Fuentes, M. D. C., Gázquez-Linares, J. J., Van Gordon, W., & Molero-Jurado, M. D. M. (2018). Effects of mindfulness training on sleep problems in patients with fibromyalgia. *Frontiers in Psychology, 9,* 1365. http://dx.doi.org/10.3389/fpsyg.2018.01365

Asmundson, G. J., & Katz, J. (2009). Understanding the co-occurrence of anxiety disorders and chronic pain: State-of-the-art. *Depression and Anxiety, 26,* 888–901. http://dx.doi.org/10.1002/da.20600

Back, S. E., Killeen, T. K., Teer, A. P., Hartwell, E. E., Federline, A., Beylotte, F., & Cox, E. Q. (2014). Substance use disorders and PTSD: An exploratory study of treatment preferences among military veterans. *Addictive Behaviors, 39,* 369–373.

Baer, R. A. (2003). Mindfulness training as a clinical intervention: A conceptual and empirical review. *Clinical Psychology: Science and Practice, 10,* 125–143. http://dx.doi.org/10.1093/clipsy.bpg015

Bair, M. J., Poleshuck, E. L., Wu, J., Krebs, E. K., Damush, T. M., Tu, W., & Kroenke, K. (2013). Anxiety but not social stressors predict 12-month depression and pain severity. *The Clinical Journal of Pain, 29,* 95–101. http://dx.doi.org/10.1097/AJP.0b013e3182652ee9

Beck, J. G., & Clapp, J. D. (2011). A different kind of comorbidity: Understanding posttraumatic stress disorder and chronic pain. *Psychological Trauma: Theory, Research, Practice, and Policy, 3,* 101–108. http://dx.doi.org/10.1037/a0021263

Bennett, H., & Wells, A. (2010). Metacognition, memory disorganization and rumination in posttraumatic stress symptoms. *Journal of Anxiety Disorders, 24,* 318–325. http://dx.doi.org/10.1016/j.janxdis.2010.01.004

Bisson, J. I., Roberts, N. P., Andrew, M., Cooper, R., & Lewis, C. (2013). Psychological therapies for chronic post-traumatic stress disorder (PTSD) in adults [Review]. *Cochrane Database of Systematic Reviews, 12,* CD003388. http://dx.doi.org/10.1002/14651858.CD003388.pub4

Boscarino, J. A. (1997). Diseases among men 20 years after exposure to severe stress: Implications for clinical research and medical care. *Psychosomatic Medicine, 59,* 605–614. http://dx.doi.org/10.1097/00006842-199711000-00008

Boscarino, J. A. (2006). Posttraumatic stress disorder and mortality among U.S. Army veterans 30 years after military service. *Annals of Epidemiology, 16,* 248–256. http://dx.doi.org/10.1016/j.annepidem.2005.03.009

Bowen, S., Chawla, N., Collins, S. E., Witkiewitz, K., Hsu, S., Grow, J., . . . Marlatt, A. (2009). Mindfulness-based relapse prevention for substance use disorders: A pilot efficacy trial. *Substance Abuse, 30,* 295–305. http://dx.doi.org/10.1080/08897070903250084

Bowen, S., Witkiewitz, K., Clifasefi, S. L., Grow, J., Chawla, N., Hsu, S. H., . . . Larimer, M. E. (2014). Relative efficacy of mindfulness-based relapse prevention, standard relapse prevention, and treatment as usual for substance use disorders: A randomized clinical trial. *JAMA Psychiatry, 71,* 547–556. http://dx.doi.org/10.1001/jamapsychiatry.2013.4546

Boyd, J. E., Lanius, R. A., & McKinnon, M. C. (2018). Mindfulness-based treatments for posttraumatic stress disorder: A review of the treatment literature and neurobiological evidence. *Journal of Psychiatry & Neuroscience, 43,* 7–25. http://dx.doi.org/10.1503/jpn.170021

Bradley, R., Greene, J., Russ, E., Dutra, L., & Westen, D. (2005). A multi-dimensional meta-analysis of psychotherapy for PTSD. *The American Journal of Psychiatry, 162*, 214–227. http://dx.doi.org/10.1176/appi.ajp.162.2.214

Bremner, J. D., Mishra, S., Campanella, C., Shah, M., Kasher, N., Evans, S., . . . Carmody, J. (2017). A pilot study of the effects of mindfulness-based stress reduction on post-traumatic stress disorder symptoms and brain response to traumatic reminders of combat in Operation Enduring Freedom/Operation Iraqi Freedom combat veterans with post-traumatic stress disorder. *Frontiers in Psychiatry, 8*, 157. Advance online publication. http://dx.doi.org/10.3389/fpsyt.2017.00157

Breslau, N., Kessler, R. C., Chilcoat, H. D., Schultz, L. R., Davis, G. C., & Andreski, P. (1998). Trauma and posttraumatic stress disorder in the community: The 1996 Detroit Area Survey of Trauma. *Archives of General Psychiatry, 55*, 626–632. http://dx.doi.org/10.1001/archpsyc.55.7.626

Brewer, J. A., Sinha, R., Chen, J. A., Michalsen, R. N., Babuscio, T. A., Nich, C., . . . Rounsaville, B. J. (2009). Mindfulness training and stress reactivity in substance abuse: Results from a randomized, controlled stage I pilot study. *Substance Abuse, 30*, 306–317. http://dx.doi.org/10.1080/08897070903250241

Briere, J. (2015). Pain and suffering: A synthesis of Buddhist and Western approaches to trauma. In V. M. Follette, J. Briere, D. Rozelle, J. W. Hopper, & D. I. Rome (Eds.), *Mindfulness-oriented interventions for trauma: Integrating contemplative practices* (pp. 11–30). New York, NY: Guilford Press.

Burton, C. (2003). Beyond somatisation: A review of the understanding and treatment of medically unexplained physical symptoms (MUPS). *British Journal of General Practice, 53*(488), 231–239.

Campbell, C. M., McCauley, L., Bounds, S. C., Mathur, V. A., Conn, L., Simango, M., . . . Fontaine, K. R. (2012). Changes in pain catastrophizing predict later changes in fibromyalgia clinical and experimental pain report: Cross-lagged panel analyses of dispositional and situational catastrophizing. *Arthritis Research & Therapy, 14*, R231. http://dx.doi.org/10.1186/ar4073

Cherkin, D. C., Sherman, K. J., Balderson, B. H., Cook, A. J., Anderson, M. L., Hawkes, R. J., . . . Turner, J. A. (2016). Effect of mindfulness-based stress reduction vs. cognitive behavioral therapy or usual care on back pain and functional limitations in adults with chronic low back pain: A randomized clinical trial. *JAMA, 315*, 1240–1249. http://dx.doi.org/10.1001/jama.2016.2323

Chesin, M. S., Benjamin-Phillips, C. A., Keilp, J., Fertuck, E. A., Brodsky, B. S., & Stanley, B. (2016). Improvements in executive attention, rumination, cognitive reactivity, and mindfulness among high-suicide risk patients participating in adjunct mindfulness-based cognitive therapy: Preliminary findings. *The Journal of Alternative and Complementary Medicine, 22*, 642–649. http://dx.doi.org/10.1089/acm.2015.0351

Chesney, E., Goodwin, G. M., & Fazel, S. (2014). Risks of all-cause and suicide mortality in mental disorders: A meta-review. *World Psychiatry, 13*, 153–160. http://dx.doi.org/10.1002/wps.20128

Chiesa, A., & Serretti, A. (2014). Are mindfulness-based interventions effective for substance use disorders? A systematic review of the evidence. *Substance Use & Misuse, 49*, 492–512. http://dx.doi.org/10.3109/10826084.2013.770027

Chopko, B. A., & Schwartz, R. C. (2013). The relation between mindfulness and posttraumatic stress symptoms among police officers. *Journal of Loss and Trauma, 18*, 1–9. http://dx.doi.org/10.1080/15325024.2012.674442

Clark, D. A., & Beck, A. T. (1990). Cognitive therapy of anxiety and depression. In R. E. Ingram (Ed.), *Contemporary psychological approaches to depression* (pp. 155–167). New York, NY: Plenum Press. http://dx.doi.org/10.1007/978-1-4613-0649-8_10

Cloitre, M. (2015). The "one size fits all" approach to trauma treatment: Should we be satisfied? *European Journal of Psychotraumatology, 6*, 27344. http://dx.doi.org/10.3402/ejpt.v6.27344

Cole, M. A., Muir, J. J., Gans, J. J., Shin, L. M., D'Esposito, M., Harel, B. T., & Schembri, A. (2015). Simultaneous treatment of neurocognitive and psychiatric symptoms in veterans with post-traumatic stress disorder and history of mild traumatic brain injury: A pilot study of mindfulness-based stress reduction. *Military Medicine, 180*, 956–963. http://dx.doi.org/10.7205/MILMED-D-14-00581

Crane, R. S., Eames, C., Kuyken, W., Hastings, R. P., Williams, J. M. G., Bartley, T., . . . Surawy, C. J. (2013). Development and validation of the mindfulness-based interventions: Teaching assessment criteria (MBI: TAC). *Assessment, 20*, 681–688. http://dx.doi.org/10.1177/1073191113490790

Crane, R. S., & Kuyken, W. (2013). The implementation of mindfulness-based cognitive therapy: Learning from the UK health service experience. *Mindfulness, 4*, 246–254. http://dx.doi.org/10.1007/s12671-012-0121-6

Crane, R. S., Kuyken, W., Hastings, R. P., Rothwell, N., & Williams, J. M. G. (2010). Training teachers to deliver mindfulness-based interventions: Learning from the UK experience. *Mindfulness, 1*, 74–86. http://dx.doi.org/10.1007/s12671-010-0010-9

Crane, R. S., Kuyken, W., Williams, J. M. G., Hastings, R. P., Cooper, L., & Fennell, M. J. V. (2012). Competence in teaching mindfulness-based courses: Concepts, development and assessment. *Mindfulness, 3*, 76–84. http://dx.doi.org/10.1007/s12671-011-0073-2

Creamer, M., Burgess, P., & McFarlane, A. C. (2001). Post-traumatic stress disorder: Findings from the Australian National Survey of Mental Health and Well-being. *Psychological Medicine, 31*, 1237–1247. http://dx.doi.org/10.1017/S0033291701004287

Creswell, J. D. (2017). Mindfulness interventions. *Annual Review of Psychology, 68*, 491–516. http://dx.doi.org/10.1146/annurev-psych-042716-051139

Crowe, M., Jordan, J., Burrell, B., Jones, V., Gillon, D., & Harris, S. (2016). Mindfulness-based stress reduction for long-term physical conditions: A systematic review. *Australian & New Zealand Journal of Psychiatry, 50*, 21–32. http://dx.doi.org/10.1177/0004867415607984

Dalgleish, T., Moradi, A. R., Taghavi, M. R., Neshat-Doost, H. T., & Yule, W. (2001). An experimental investigation of hypervigilance for threat in children and adolescents with post-traumatic stress disorder. *Psychological Medicine, 31*, 541–547. http://dx.doi.org/10.1017/S0033291701003567

Davidson, J. R. T. (2001). Recognition and treatment of posttraumatic stress disorder. *JAMA, 286*, 584–588. http://dx.doi.org/10.1001/jama.286.5.584

Davis, D. A., Luecken, L. J., & Zautra, A. J. (2005). Are reports of childhood abuse related to the experience of chronic pain in adulthood? A meta-analytic review of the literature. *The Clinical Journal of Pain, 21*, 398–405. http://dx.doi.org/10.1097/01.ajp.0000149795.08746.31

Davis, L. L., Whetsell, C., Hamner, M. B., Carmody, J., Rothbaum, B. O., Allen, R. S., . . . Bremner, J. D. (2018). A multisite randomized controlled trial of mindfulness-based stress reduction in the treatment of posttraumatic stress disorder. *Psychiatric Research & Clinical Practice.* Advance online publication. Retrieved from http://dx.doi.org/10.1176/appi.prcp.20180002

Day, M. A. (2017). *Mindfulness-based cognitive therapy for chronic pain: A clinical manual and guide.* Malden, MA: Wiley. http://dx.doi.org/10.1002/9781119257875

Day, M. A., Jensen, M. P., Ehde, D. M., & Thorn, B. E. (2014). Toward a theoretical model for mindfulness-based pain management. *The Journal of Pain, 15*, 691–703. http://dx.doi.org/10.1016/j.jpain.2014.03.003

Deyo, M., Wilson, K. A., Ong, J., & Koopman, C. (2009). Mindfulness and rumination: Does mindfulness training lead to reductions in the ruminative thinking associated with depression? *EXPLORE: The Journal of Science and Healing, 5*, 265–271. http://dx.doi.org/10.1016/j.explore.2009.06.005

Dobie, D. J., Kivlahan, D. R., Maynard, C., Bush, K. R., Davis, T. M., & Bradley, K. A. (2004). Posttraumatic stress disorder in female veterans: Association with self-reported health problems and functional impairment. *Archives of Internal Medicine, 164*, 394–400. http://dx.doi.org/10.1001/archinte.164.4.394

Dorado, K., Schreiber, K. L., Koulouris, A., Edwards, R. R., Napadow, V., & Lazaridou, A. (2018). Interactive effects of pain catastrophizing and mindfulness on pain intensity in women with fibromyalgia. *Health Psychology Open, 5.* http://dx.doi.org/10.1177/2055102918807406

Dorrepaal, E., Thomaes, K., Hoogendoorn, A. W., Veltman, D. J., Draijer, N., & van Balkom, A. J. (2014). Evidence-based treatment for adult women with child abuse-related complex PTSD: A quantitative review. *European Journal of Psychotraumatology, 5*, 23613. http://dx.doi.org/10.3402/ejpt.v5.23613

Drossman, D. A. (2016). Functional gastrointestinal disorders: History, pathophysiology, clinical features, and Rome IV. *Gastroenterology, 150*, 1262–1279e2. http://dx.doi.org/10.1053/j.gastro.2016.02.032

Drossman, D. A., Leserman, J., Li, Z., Keefe, F., Hu, Y. J., & Toomey, T. C. (2000). Effects of coping on health outcome among women with gastrointestinal disorders. *Psychosomatic Medicine, 62*, 309–317. http://dx.doi.org/10.1097/00006842-200005000-00004

Duncan, L. G., & Bardacke, N. (2010). Mindfulness-based childbirth and parenting education: Promoting family mindfulness during the perinatal period. *Journal of Child and Family Studies, 19,* 190–202. http://dx.doi.org/10.1007/s10826-009-9313-7

Dutton, M. A. (2015). Mindfulness-based stress reduction for underserved trauma populations. In V. Follette, J. Briere, D. Rozelle, J. W. Hopper, & D. I. Rome (Eds.), *Mindfulness-oriented interventions for trauma* (pp. 243–256). New York, NY: Guilford Press.

Dutton, M. A., Bermudez, D., Matás, A., Majid, H., & Myers, N. L. (2013). Mindfulness-based stress reduction for low-income, predominantly African American women with PTSD and a history of intimate partner violence. *Cognitive and Behavioral Practice, 20,* 23–32. http://dx.doi.org/10.1016/j.cbpra.2011.08.003

Ehlers, A., & Clark, D. M. (2000). A cognitive model of posttraumatic stress disorder. *Behaviour Research and Therapy, 38,* 319–345. http://dx.doi.org/10.1016/S0005-7967(99)00123-0

Ehring, T., Szeimies, A.-K., & Schaffrick, C. (2009). An experimental analogue study into the role of abstract thinking in trauma-related rumination. *Behaviour Research and Therapy, 47,* 285–293. http://dx.doi.org/10.1016/j.brat.2008.12.011

Eisendrath, S. J., Gillung, E., Delucchi, K., Mathalon, D. H., Yang, T. T., Satre, D. D., . . . Wolkowitz, O. M. (2015). A preliminary study: Efficacy of mindfulness-based cognitive therapy versus sertraline as first-line treatments for major depressive disorder. *Mindfulness, 6,* 475–482. http://dx.doi.org/10.1007/s12671-014-0280-8

Engler, J. (2006). Promises and perils of the spiritual path. In M. Unno (Ed.), *Buddhism and psychotherapy across cultures: Essays on theories and practices* (pp. 17–30). Somerville, MA: Wisdom.

Epstein, M. A. (2013). *The trauma of everyday life.* London, England: Penguin Books.

Erbes, C. R., Thuras, P., Lim, K. O., & Polusny, M. A. (2017). Letter in response to Drs. Lee and Hoge's commentary. *Evidence-Based Mental Health, 20,* 31. http://dx.doi.org/10.1136/eb-2016-102595

Felleman, B. I., Stewart, D. G., Simpson, T. L., Heppner, P. S., & Kearney, D. J. (2016). Predictors of depression and PTSD treatment response among veterans participating in mindfulness-based stress reduction. *Mindfulness, 7,* 886–895. http://dx.doi.org/10.1007/s12671-016-0527-7

Foa, E. B., & Kozak, M. J. (1986). Emotional processing of fear: Exposure to corrective information. *Psychological Bulletin, 99,* 20–35.

Foa, E. B., & Riggs, D. S. (1993). Posttraumatic stress disorder and rape. *American Psychiatric Press Review of Psychiatry, 12,* 273–303.

Fresco, D. M., Moore, M. T., van Dulmen, M. H. M., Segal, Z. V., Ma, S. H., Teasdale, J. D., & Williams, J. M. G. (2007). Initial psychometric properties of the Experiences Questionnaire: Validation of a self-report measure of decentering. *Behavior Therapy, 38,* 234–246. http://dx.doi.org/10.1016/j.beth.2006.08.003

Frewen, P. A., Dozois, D. J. A., Neufeld, R. W. J., & Lanius, R. A. (2012). Disturbances of emotional awareness and expression in posttraumatic stress disorder: Meta-mood, emotion regulation, mindfulness, and interference of emotional expressiveness. *Psychological Trauma: Theory, Research, Practice, and Policy, 4,* 152–161. http://dx.doi.org/10.1037/a0023114

Friedman, M. J., Resick, P. A., & Keane, T. M. (2014). *Handbook of PTSD: Science and practice* (2nd ed.). New York, NY: Guilford Press.

Frost, N. D., Laska, K. M., & Wampold, B. E. (2014). The evidence for present-centered therapy as a treatment for posttraumatic stress disorder. *Journal of Traumatic Stress, 27,* 1–8. http://dx.doi.org/10.1002/jts.21881

Gallegos, A. M., Crean, H. F., Pigeon, W. R., & Heffner, K. L. (2017). Meditation and yoga for posttraumatic stress disorder: A meta-analytic review of randomized controlled trials. *Clinical Psychology Review, 58,* 115–124. http://dx.doi.org/10.1016/j.cpr.2017.10.004

Garland, E. L., & Howard, M. O. (2018). Mindfulness-based treatment of addiction: Current state of the field and envisioning the next wave of research. *Addiction Science & Clinical Practice, 13,* 14. http://dx.doi.org/10.1186/s13722-018-0115-3

Gerlock, A. A., Grimesey, J., & Sayre, G. (2014). Military-related posttraumatic stress disorder and intimate relationship behaviors: A developing dyadic relationship model. *Journal of Marital and Family Therapy, 40,* 344–356. http://dx.doi.org/10.1111/jmft.12017

Gilbert, P., & Procter, S. (2006). Compassionate mind training for people with high shame and self-criticism: Overview and pilot study of a group therapy approach. *Clinical Psychology & Psychotherapy, 13,* 353–379. http://dx.doi.org/10.1002/cpp.507

Goldberg, S. B., Tucker, R. P., Greene, P. A., Davidson, R. J., Kearney, D. J., & Simpson, T. L. (2019). Mindfulness-based cognitive therapy for the treatment of current depressive symptoms: A meta-analysis. *Cognitive Behaviour Therapy.* http://dx.doi.org/10.1080/16506073.2018.1556330

Goldberg, S. B., Tucker, R. P., Greene, P. A., Davidson, R. J., Wampold, B. E., Kearney, D. J., & Simpson, T. L. (2018). Mindfulness-based interventions for psychiatric disorders: A systematic review and meta-analysis. *Clinical Psychology Review, 59,* 52–60. http://dx.doi.org/10.1016/j.cpr.2017.10.011

Goldberg, S. B., Tucker, R. P., Greene, P. A., Simpson, T. L., Kearney, D. J., & Davidson, R. J. (2017). Is mindfulness research methodology improving over time? A systematic review. *PLoS ONE, 12,* e0187298. http://dx.doi.org/10.1371/journal.pone.0187298

Goldsmith, R. E., Gerhart, J. I., Chesney, S. A., Burns, J. W., Kleinman, B., & Hood, M. M. (2014). Mindfulness-based stress reduction for posttraumatic stress symptoms: Building acceptance and decreasing shame. *Journal of Evidence-Based Complementary & Alternative Medicine, 19*, 227–234.

Goldstein, R. B., Smith, S. M., Chou, S. P., Saha, T. D., Jung, J., Zhang, H., . . . Grant, B. F. (2016). The epidemiology of *DSM–5* posttraumatic stress disorder in the United States: Results from the National Epidemiologic Survey on Alcohol and Related Conditions-III. *Social Psychiatry and Psychiatric Epidemiology, 51*, 1137–1148. http://dx.doi.org/10.1007/s00127-016-1208-5

Goyal, M., Singh, S., Sibinga, E. M., Gould, N. F., Rowland-Seymour, A., Sharma, R., . . . Haythornthwaite, J. A. (2014). Meditation programs for psychological stress and well-being: A systematic review and meta-analysis. *JAMA Internal Medicine, 174*, 357–368. http://dx.doi.org/10.1001/jamainternmed.2013.13018

Grabovac, A. D., Lau, M. A., & Willett, B. R. (2011). Mechanisms of mindfulness: A Buddhist psychological model. *Mindfulness, 2*, 154–166. http://dx.doi.org/10.1007/s12671-011-0054-5

Harding, K., Simpson, T., & Kearney, D. J. (2018). Reduced symptoms of post-traumatic stress disorder and irritable bowel syndrome following mindfulness-based stress reduction among veterans. *The Journal of Alternative and Complementary Medicine, 24*, 1159–1165. http://dx.doi.org/10.1089/acm.2018.0135

Hayes, S. C., Strosahl, K., & Wilson, K. G. (1999). *Acceptance and commitment therapy: An experiential approach to behavior change.* New York, NY: Guilford Press.

Hilton, L., Ruelaz Maher, A., Colaiaco, B., Apaydin, E., Sorbero, M., Booth, M., . . . Hempel, S. (2016). Meditation for posttraumatic stress: Systematic review and meta-analysis. *Psychological Trauma: Theory, Research, Practice, and Policy, 9*, 453–460. http://dx.doi.org/10.1037/tra0000180

Hofmann, S. G., Sawyer, A. T., Witt, A. A., & Oh, D. (2010). The effect of mindfulness-based therapy on anxiety and depression: A meta-analytic review. *Journal of Consulting and Clinical Psychology, 78*, 169–183. http://dx.doi.org/10.1037/a0018555

Holliday, S. B., Hull, A., Lockwood, C., Eickhoff, C., Sullivan, P., & Reinhard, M. (2014). Physical health, mental health, and utilization of complementary and alternative medicine services among Gulf War veterans. *Medical Care, 52*(Suppl. 5), S39–S44. http://dx.doi.org/10.1097/MLR.0000000000000223

Hölzel, B. K., Lazar, S. W., Gard, T., Schuman-Olivier, Z., Vago, D. R., & Ott, U. (2011). How does mindfulness meditation work? Proposing mechanisms of action from a conceptual and neural perspective. *Perspectives on Psychological Science, 6*, 537–559. http://dx.doi.org/10.1177/1745691611419671

Huijbers, M. J., Spinhoven, P., Spijker, J., Ruhé, H. G., van Schaik, D. J., van Oppen, P., . . . Speckens, A. E. (2016). Discontinuation of antidepressant medication after mindfulness-based cognitive therapy for recurrent depression: Randomised controlled non-inferiority trial. *The British Journal of Psychiatry, 208*, 366–373. http://dx.doi.org/10.1192/bjp.bp.115.168971

Hundt, N. E., Harik, J. M., Thompson, K. E., Barrera, T. L., & Miles, S. R. (2018). Increased utilization of prolonged exposure and cognitive processing therapy over time: A case example from a large Veterans Affairs posttraumatic stress disorder clinic. *Psychological Services, 15*, 429–436. http://dx.doi.org/10.1037/ser0000138

Imel, Z. E., Laska, K., Jakupcak, M., & Simpson, T. L. (2013). Meta-analysis of dropout in treatments for posttraumatic stress disorder. *Journal of Consulting and Clinical Psychology, 81*, 394–404. http://dx.doi.org/10.1037/a0031474

Jain, S., Shapiro, S. L., Swanick, S., Roesch, S. C., Mills, P. J., Bell, I., & Schwartz, G. E. R. (2007). A randomized controlled trial of mindfulness meditation versus relaxation training: Effects on distress, positive states of mind, rumination, and distraction. *Annals of Behavioral Medicine, 33*, 11–21. http://dx.doi.org/10.1207/s15324796abm3301_2

Jakupcak, M., Hoerster, K. D., Varra, A., Vannoy, S., Felker, B., & Hunt, S. (2011). Hopelessness and suicidal ideation in Iraq and Afghanistan War veterans reporting subthreshold and threshold posttraumatic stress disorder. *Journal of Nervous and Mental Disease, 199*, 272–275. http://dx.doi.org/10.1097/NMD.0b013e3182124604

Jeffreys, M. D., Reinfeld, C., Nair, P. V., Garcia, H. A., Mata-Galan, E., & Rentz, T. O. (2014). Evaluating treatment of posttraumatic stress disorder with cognitive processing therapy and prolonged exposure therapy in a VHA specialty clinic. *Journal of Anxiety Disorders, 28*, 108–114. http://dx.doi.org/10.1016/j.janxdis.2013.04.010

Jensen, M. P. (2011). Psychosocial approaches to pain management: An organizational framework. *Pain, 152*, 717–725. http://dx.doi.org/10.1016/j.pain.2010.09.002

Kabat-Zinn, J. (1982). An outpatient program in behavioral medicine for chronic pain patients based on the practice of mindfulness meditation: Theoretical considerations and preliminary results. *General Hospital Psychiatry, 4*, 33–47. http://dx.doi.org/10.1016/0163-8343(82)90026-3

Kabat-Zinn, J. (2005). *Full catastrophe living: Using the wisdom of your body and mind to face stress, pain, and illness* (15th ann. ed.). New York, NY: Delta Trade Paperback/Bantam Dell.

Kabat-Zinn, J. (2009). *Full catastrophe living: Using the wisdom of your body and mind to face stress, pain, and illness*. New York, NY: Delta.

Kabat-Zinn, J. (2013). *Full catastrophe living: Using the wisdom of your body and mind to face stress, pain, and illness* (2nd ed.). New York, NY: Bantam Books.

Kabat-Zinn, J., Lipworth, L., Burncy, R., & Sellers, W. (1986). Four-year follow-up of a meditation-based program for the self-regulation of chronic pain: Treatment outcomes and compliance. *The Clinical Journal of Pain, 2*, 159–173. http://dx.doi.org/10.1097/00002508-198602030-00004

Kamenov, K., Mellor-Marsá, B., Leal, I., Ayuso-Mateos, J. L., & Cabello, M. (2014). Analysing psychosocial difficulties in depression: A content comparison between systematic literature review and patient perspective. *BioMed*

Research International, 2014, 319634. Advance online publication. http://dx.doi.org/10.1155/2014/319634

Karam, E. G., Friedman, M. J., Hill, E. D., Kessler, R. C., McLaughlin, K. A., Petukhova, M., . . . Koenen, K. C. (2014). Cumulative traumas and risk thresholds: 12-month PTSD in the World Mental Health (WMH) surveys. *Depression and Anxiety, 31,* 130–142. http://dx.doi.org/10.1002/da.22169

Kazdin, A. E., & Nock, M. K. (2003). Delineating mechanisms of change in child and adolescent therapy: Methodological issues and research recommendations. *The Journal of Child Psychology and Psychiatry, 44,* 1116–1129. http://dx.doi.org/10.1111/1469-7610.00195

Kearney, D. J., Malte, C. A., McManus, C., Martinez, M. E., Felleman, B., & Simpson, T. L. (2013). Loving-kindness meditation for posttraumatic stress disorder: A pilot study. *Journal of Traumatic Stress, 26,* 426–434. http://dx.doi.org/10.1002/jts.21832

Kearney, D. J., McDermott, K., Malte, C., Martinez, M., & Simpson, T. L. (2012). Association of participation in a mindfulness program with measures of PTSD, depression and quality of life in a veteran sample. *Journal of Clinical Psychology, 68,* 101–116. http://dx.doi.org/10.1002/jclp.20853

Kearney, D. J., McDermott, K., Malte, C., Martinez, M., & Simpson, T. L. (2013). Effects of participation in a mindfulness program for veterans with posttraumatic stress disorder: A randomized controlled pilot study. *Journal of Clinical Psychology, 69,* 14–27. http://dx.doi.org/10.1002/jclp.21911

Kearney, D. J., McManus, C., Malte, C. A., Martinez, M., Felleman, B. I., & Simpson, T. (2014). Loving-kindness meditation and the broaden-and-build theory of positive emotions among veterans with posttraumatic stress disorder. *Medical Care, 52*(Suppl. 6), S32–S38.

Kearney, D. J., & Simpson, T. L. (2015). Broadening the approach to posttraumatic stress disorder and the consequences of trauma. *JAMA, 314,* 453–455. http://dx.doi.org/10.1001/jama.2015.7522

Kearney, D. J., Simpson, T. L., Malte, C. A., Felleman, B., Martinez, M. E., & Hunt, S. C. (2016). Mindfulness-based stress reduction in addition to usual care is associated with improvements in pain, fatigue, and cognitive failures among veterans with Gulf War illness. *The American Journal of Medicine, 129,* 204–214. http://dx.doi.org/10.1016/j.amjmed.2015.09.015

Kehle-Forbes, S. M., Meis, L. A., Spoont, M. R., & Polusny, M. A. (2016). Treatment initiation and dropout from prolonged exposure and cognitive processing therapy in a VA outpatient clinic. *Psychological Trauma: Theory, Research, Practice, and Policy, 8,* 107–114. http://dx.doi.org/10.1037/tra0000065

Kessler, R. C. (2000). Posttraumatic stress disorder: The burden to the individual and to society. *The Journal of Clinical Psychiatry, 61*(Suppl. 5), 4–12.

Kessler, R. C., Berglund, P., Demler, O., Jin, R., Merikangas, K. R., & Walters, E. E. (2005). Lifetime prevalence and age-of-onset distributions of DSM-IV disorders in the National Comorbidity Survey replication: Erratum. *Archives of General Psychiatry, 62,* 768. http://dx.doi.org/10.1001/archpsyc.62.7.768

Kessler, R. C., Borges, G., & Walters, E. E. (1999). Prevalence of and risk factors for lifetime suicide attempts in the National Comorbidity Survey. *Archives of General Psychiatry, 56*, 617–626. http://dx.doi.org/10.1001/archpsyc.56.7.617

Kessler, R. C., Sonnega, A., Bromet, E., Hughes, M., & Nelson, C. B. (1995). Posttraumatic stress disorder in the national comorbidity survey. *Archives of General Psychiatry, 52*, 1048–1060. http://dx.doi.org/10.1001/archpsyc.1995.03950240066012

Khantzian, E. J. (2003). The self-medication hypothesis revisited: The dually diagnosed patient. *Primary Psychiatry, 10*(9), 47–54.

Kimbrough, E., Magyari, T., Langenberg, P., Chesney, M., & Berman, B. (2010). Mindfulness intervention for child abuse survivors. *Journal of Clinical Psychology, 66*, 17–33. http://dx.doi.org/10.1002/jclp.20624

King, A. P., Block, S. R., Sripada, R. K., Rauch, S., Giardino, N., Favorite, T., . . . Liberzon, I. (2016). Altered default mode network (DMN) resting state functional connectivity following a mindfulness-based exposure therapy for posttraumatic stress disorder (PTSD) in combat veterans of Afghanistan and Iraq. *Depression and Anxiety, 33*, 289–299. http://dx.doi.org/10.1002/da.22481

King, A. P., Erickson, T. M., Giardino, N. D., Favorite, T., Rauch, S. A., Robinson, E., . . . Liberzon, I. (2013). A pilot study of group mindfulness-based cognitive therapy (MBCT) for combat veterans with posttraumatic stress disorder (PTSD). *Depression and Anxiety, 30*, 638–645. http://dx.doi.org/10.1002/da.22104

Kingston, T., Dooley, B., Bates, A., Lawlor, E., & Malone, K. (2007). Mindfulness-based cognitive therapy for residual depressive symptoms. *Psychology and Psychotherapy: Theory, Research and Practice, 80*, 193–203. http://dx.doi.org/10.1348/147608306X116016

Koob, G. F., & Volkow, N. D. (2010). Neurocircuitry of addiction. *Neuropsychopharmacology, 35*, 217–238. http://dx.doi.org/10.1038/npp.2009.110

Kornfield, J. (1993). *A path with heart*. New York, NY: Bantam.

Kraemer, H. C., Wilson, G. T., Fairburn, C. G., & Agras, W. S. (2002). Mediators and moderators of treatment effects in randomized clinical trials. *Archives of General Psychiatry, 59*, 877–883. http://dx.doi.org/10.1001/archpsyc.59.10.877

Krejci, L. P., Carter, K., & Gaudet, T. (2014). Whole health: The vision and implementation of personalized, proactive, patient-driven health care for veterans. *Medical Care, 52*(Suppl. 5), S5–S8. http://dx.doi.org/10.1097/MLR.0000000000000226

Kristeller, J., Wolever, R. Q., & Sheets, V. (2014). Mindfulness-based eating awareness training (MB-EAT) for binge eating: A randomized clinical trial. *Mindfulness, 5*, 282–297. http://dx.doi.org/10.1007/s12671-012-0179-1

Kroenke, K., Wu, J., Bair, M. J., Krebs, E. E., Damush, T. M., & Tu, W. (2011). Reciprocal relationship between pain and depression: A 12-month longitudinal analysis in primary care. *The Journal of Pain, 12*, 964–973. http://dx.doi.org/10.1016/j.jpain.2011.03.003

Kroesen, K., Baldwin, C. M., Brooks, A. J., & Bell, I. R. (2002). US military veterans' perceptions of the conventional medical care system and their use of complementary and alternative medicine. *Family Practice, 19*, 57–64. http://dx.doi.org/10.1093/fampra/19.1.57

Kummar, A. S. (2018). Mindfulness and fear extinction: A brief review of its current neuropsychological literature and possible implications for posttraumatic stress disorder. *Psychological Reports, 121*, 792–814.

Kuyken, W., Hayes, R., Barrett, B., Byng, R., Dalgleish, T., Kessler, D., . . . Byford, S. (2015). Effectiveness and cost-effectiveness of mindfulness-based cognitive therapy compared with maintenance antidepressant treatment in the prevention of depressive relapse or recurrence (PREVENT): A randomised controlled trial. *The Lancet, 386*, 63–73. http://dx.doi.org/10.1016/S0140-6736(14)62222-4

Kuyken, W., Warren, F. C., Taylor, R. S., Whalley, B., Crane, C., Bondolfi, G., . . . Dalgleish, T. (2016). Efficacy of mindfulness-based cognitive therapy in prevention of depressive relapse: An individual patient data meta-analysis from randomized trials. *JAMA Psychiatry, 73*, 565–574. http://dx.doi.org/10.1001/jamapsychiatry.2016.0076

Kuyken, W., Watkins, E., Holden, E., White, K., Taylor, R. S., Byford, S., . . . Dalgleish, T. (2010). How does mindfulness-based cognitive therapy work? *Behaviour Research and Therapy, 48*, 1105–1112. http://dx.doi.org/10.1016/j.brat.2010.08.003

Lacy, B. E., & Patel, N. K. (2017). Rome criteria and a diagnostic approach to irritable bowel syndrome. *Journal of Clinical Medicine, 6*, 99. http://dx.doi.org/10.3390/jcm6110099

Lakhan, S. E., & Schofield, K. L. (2013). Mindfulness-based therapies in the treatment of somatization disorders: A systematic review and meta-analysis. *PLoS ONE, 8*, e71834. http://dx.doi.org/10.1371/journal.pone.0071834

Lang, A. J., Strauss, J. L., Bomyea, J., Bormann, J. E., Hickman, S. D., Good, R. C., & Essex, M. (2012). The theoretical and empirical basis for meditation as an intervention for PTSD. *Behavior Modification, 36*, 759–786. Advance online publication. http://dx.doi.org/10.1177/0145445512441200

Lee, D. A., Scragg, P., & Turner, S. (2001). The role of shame and guilt in traumatic events: A clinical model of shame-based and guilt-based PTSD. *British Journal of Medical Psychology, 74*, 451–466.

Lee, D. J., & Hoge, C. W. (2017). Significant methodological flaws limit conclusions drawn by authors of a recent PTSD mindfulness study. *Evidence-Based Mental Health, 20*, 30. http://dx.doi.org/10.1136/eb-2016-102308

Li, W., Howard, M. O., Garland, E. L., McGovern, P., & Lazar, M. (2017). Mindfulness treatment for substance misuse: A systematic review and meta-analysis. *Journal of Substance Abuse Treatment, 75*, 62–96. http://dx.doi.org/10.1016/j.jsat.2017.01.008

Libby, D. J., Pilver, C. E., & Desai, R. (2012). Complementary and alternative medicine in VA specialized PTSD treatment programs. *Psychiatric Services, 63*, 1134–1136. http://dx.doi.org/10.1176/appi.ps.201100456

Libby, D. J., Pilver, C. E., & Desai, R. (2013). Complementary and alternative medicine use among individuals with posttraumatic stress disorder. *Psychological Trauma: Theory, Research, Practice, and Policy, 5*, 277–285. http://dx.doi.org/10.1037/a0027082

Litz, B. T., & Gray, M. J. (2002). Emotional numbing in posttraumatic stress disorder: Current and future research directions. *Australian & New Zealand Journal of Psychiatry, 36*, 198–204. http://dx.doi.org/10.1046/j.1440-1614.2002.01002.x

Lucey, B. P., Clifford, D. B., Creighton, J., Edwards, R. R., McArthur, J. C., & Haythornthwaite, J. (2011). Relationship of depression and catastrophizing to pain, disability, and medication adherence in patients with HIV-associated sensory neuropathy. *AIDS Care, 23*, 921–928. http://dx.doi.org/10.1080/09540121.2010.543883

Lynch, T. R., Chapman, A. L., Rosenthal, M. Z., Kuo, J. R., & Linehan, M. M. (2006). Mechanisms of change in dialectical behavior therapy: Theoretical and empirical observations. *Journal of Clinical Psychology, 62*, 459–480. http://dx.doi.org/10.1002/jclp.20243

Ma, S. H., & Teasdale, J. D. (2004). Mindfulness-based cognitive therapy for depression: Replication and exploration of differential relapse prevention effects. *Journal of Consulting and Clinical Psychology, 72*, 31–40. http://dx.doi.org/10.1037/0022-006X.72.1.31

Maguen, S., Madden, E., Cohen, B., Bertenthal, D., & Seal, K. (2014). Association of mental health problems with gastrointestinal disorders in Iraq and Afghanistan veterans. *Depression and Anxiety, 31*, 160–165. http://dx.doi.org/10.1002/da.22072

Magyari, T. (2015). Teaching mindfulness-based stress reduction and mindfulness to women with complex trauma. In V. Follette, J. Briere, D. Rozelle, J. W. Hopper, & D. I. Rome (Eds.), *Mindfulness-oriented interventions for trauma* (pp. 140–156). New York, NY: Guilford Press.

Markowitz, J. C., Petkova, E., Neria, Y., Van Meter, P. E., Zhao, Y., Hembree, E., . . . Marshall, R. D. (2015). Is exposure necessary? A randomized clinical trial of interpersonal psychotherapy for PTSD. *The American Journal of Psychiatry, 172*, 430–440. http://dx.doi.org/10.1176/appi.ajp.2014.14070908

Martinez, M. E., Kearney, D. J., Simpson, T., Felleman, B. I., Bernardi, N., & Sayre, G. (2015). Challenges to enrollment and participation in mindfulness-based stress reduction among veterans: A qualitative study. *The Journal of Alternative and Complementary Medicine, 21*, 409–421. http://dx.doi.org/10.1089/acm.2014.0324

Meichenbaum, D. (2007). Stress inoculation training: A preventative and treatment approach. In P. M. Lehrer, R. L. Woolfolk, & W. S. Sime (Eds.), *Principles and practice of stress management* (3rd ed.; pp. 497–518). New York, NY: Guilford Press.

Meichenbaum, D. (2017). Stress inoculation training: A preventative and treatment approach. In D. Meichenbaum (Ed.), *The evolution of cognitive behavior therapy* (pp. 101–124). New York, NY: Routledge. http://dx.doi.org/10.4324/9781315748931

Mindfulness All-Party Parliamentary Group. (2015). *Mindful nation UK: Report by the Mindfulness All-Party Parliamentary Group (MAPPG)*. Sheffield, England: Author.

Moore, K. M., & Martin, M. E. (2015). Using MBCT in a chronic pain setting: A qualitative analysis of participants' experiences. *Mindfulness, 6*, 1129–1136.

Müller-Engelmann, M., Wünsch, S., Volk, M., & Steil, R. (2017). Mindfulness-based stress reduction (MBSR) as a standalone intervention for posttraumatic stress disorder after mixed traumatic events: A mixed-methods feasibility study. *Frontiers in Psychology, 8*, 1407. Advance online publication. http://dx.doi.org/10.3389/fpsyg.2017.01407

Neff, K. D., & Germer, C. K. (2013). A pilot study and randomized controlled trial of the mindful self-compassion program. *Journal of Clinical Psychology, 69*, 28–44.

Niles, B. L., Klunk-Gillis, J., Ryngala, D. J., Silberbogen, A. K., Paysnick, A., & Wolf, E. J. (2012). Comparing mindfulness and psychoeducation treatments for combat-related PTSD using a telehealth approach. *Psychological Trauma: Theory, Research, Practice, and Policy, 4*, 538–547. http://dx.doi.org/10.1037/a0026161

Niles, B. L., Mori, D. L., Polizzi, C., Pless Kaiser, A., Weinstein, E. S., Gershkovich, M., & Wang, C. (2018). A systematic review of randomized trials of mind-body interventions for PTSD. *Journal of Clinical Psychology, 74*, 1485–1508. http://dx.doi.org/10.1002/jclp.22634

Nock, M. K. (2007). Conceptual and design essentials for evaluating mechanisms of change. *Alcoholism: Clinical & Experimental Research, 31*, 4s–12s. http://dx.doi.org/10.1111/j.1530-0277.2007.00488.x

Nolen-Hoeksema, S. (1991). Responses to depression and their effects on the duration of depressive episodes. *Journal of Abnormal Psychology, 100*, 569–582. http://dx.doi.org/10.1037/0021-843X.100.4.569

Nolen-Hoeksema, S. (2000). The role of rumination in depressive disorders and mixed anxiety/depressive symptoms. *Journal of Abnormal Psychology, 109*, 504–511. http://dx.doi.org/10.1037/0021-843X.109.3.504

Norman, S. B., Haller, M., Kim, H. M., Allard, C. B., Porter, K. E., Stein, M. B., . . . Rauch, S. A. M. (2018). Trauma related guilt cognitions partially mediate the relationship between PTSD symptom severity and functioning among returning combat veterans. *Journal of Psychiatric Research, 100*, 56–62. http://dx.doi.org/10.1016/j.jpsychires.2018.02.003

Norris, F. H., Murphy, A. D., Baker, C. K., & Perilla, J. L. (2003). Severity, timing, and duration of reactions to trauma in the population: An example from Mexico. *Biological Psychiatry, 53*, 769–778. http://dx.doi.org/10.1016/S0006-3223(03)00086-6

Olatunji, B. O., Cisler, J. M., & Tolin, D. F. (2007). Quality of life in the anxiety disorders: A meta-analytic review. *Clinical Psychology Review, 27*, 572–581. http://dx.doi.org/10.1016/j.cpr.2007.01.015

Otis, J. D., Gregor, K., Hardway, C., Morrison, J., Scioli, E., & Sanderson, K. (2010). An examination of the co-morbidity between chronic pain and posttraumatic stress disorder on U.S. veterans. *Psychological Services, 7*, 126–135. http://dx.doi.org/10.1037/a0020512

Palmer, P. J. (2009). *A hidden wholeness: The journey toward an undivided life.* San Francisco, CA: Wiley.

Palpacuer, C., Gallet, L., Drapier, D., Reymann, J.-M., Falissard, B., & Naudet, F. (2017). Specific and non-specific effects of psychotherapeutic interventions for depression: Results from a meta-analysis of 84 studies. *Journal of Psychiatric Research, 87*, 95–104. http://dx.doi.org/10.1016/j.jpsychires.2016.12.015

Panagioti, M., Gooding, P. A., & Tarrier, N. (2012). A meta-analysis of the association between posttraumatic stress disorder and suicidality: The role of comorbid depression. *Comprehensive Psychiatry, 53*, 915–930. http://dx.doi.org/10.1016/j.comppsych.2012.02.009

Piet, J., & Hougaard, E. (2011). The effect of mindfulness-based cognitive therapy for prevention of relapse in recurrent major depressive disorder: A systematic review and meta-analysis. *Clinical Psychology Review, 31*, 1032–1040. http://dx.doi.org/10.1016/j.cpr.2011.05.002

Pole, N., Neylan, T. C., Otte, C., Metzler, T. J., Best, S. R., Henn-Haase, C., & Marmar, C. (2007). Associations between childhood trauma and emotion-modulated psychophysiological responses to startling sounds: A study of police cadets. *116*, 352–361. http://dx.doi.org/10.1037/0021-843X.116.2.352

Polusny, M. A., Erbes, C. R., Thuras, P., Moran, A., Lamberty, G. J., Collins, R. C., . . . Lim, K. O. (2015). Mindfulness-based stress reduction for posttraumatic stress disorder among veterans: A randomized clinical trial. *JAMA, 314*, 456–465. http://dx.doi.org/10.1001/jama.2015.8361

Possemato, K., Bergen-Cico, D., Treatman, S., Allen, C., Wade, M., & Pigeon, W. (2016). A randomized clinical trial of primary care brief mindfulness training for veterans with PTSD. *Journal of Clinical Psychology, 72*, 179–193. http://dx.doi.org/10.1002/jclp.22241

Power, M. J., & Fyvie, C. (2013). The role of emotion in PTSD: Two preliminary studies. *Behavioural and Cognitive Psychotherapy, 41*, 162–172. http://dx.doi.org/10.1017/S1352465812000148

Powers, M. B., Halpern, J. M., Ferenschak, M. P., Gillihan, S. J., & Foa, E. B. (2010). A meta-analytic review of prolonged exposure for posttraumatic stress disorder. *Clinical Psychology Review, 30*, 635–641. http://dx.doi.org/10.1016/j.cpr.2010.04.007

Ramel, W. I., Goldin, P. R., Carmona, P. E., & McQuaid, J. R. (2004). The effects of mindfulness meditation on cognitive processes and affect in patients with past depression. *Cognitive Therapy and Research, 28*, 433–455. http://dx.doi.org/10.1023/B:COTR.0000045557.15923.96

Rapaport, M. H., Clary, C., Fayyad, R., & Endicott, J. (2005). Quality-of-life impairment in depressive and anxiety disorders. *The American Journal of Psychiatry, 162*, 1171–1178. http://dx.doi.org/10.1176/appi.ajp.162.6.1171

Reiner, K., Tibi, L., & Lipsitz, J. D. (2013). Do mindfulness-based interventions reduce pain intensity? A critical review of the literature. *Pain Medicine, 14,* 230–242. http://dx.doi.org/10.1111/pme.12006

Resick, P. A., & Miller, M. W. (2009). Posttraumatic stress disorder: Anxiety or traumatic stress disorder? *Journal of Traumatic Stress, 22,* 384–390. http://dx.doi.org/10.1002/jts.20437

Resick, P. A., Wachen, J. S., Mintz, J., Young-McCaughan, S., Roache, J. D., Borah, A. M., . . . Peterson, A. L. (2015). A randomized clinical trial of group cognitive processing therapy compared with group present-centered therapy for PTSD among active duty military personnel. *Journal of Consulting and Clinical Psychology, 83,* 1058–1068. http://dx.doi.org/10.1037/ccp0000016

Resick, P. A., Williams, L. F., Suvak, M. K., Monson, C. M., & Gradus, J. L. (2012). Long-term outcomes of cognitive–behavioral treatments for posttraumatic stress disorder among female rape survivors. *Journal of Consulting and Clinical Psychology, 80,* 201–210. http://dx.doi.org/10.1037/a0026602

Rimes, K. A., & Wingrove, J. (2013). Mindfulness-based cognitive therapy for people with chronic fatigue syndrome still experiencing excessive fatigue after cognitive behaviour therapy: A pilot randomized study. *Clinical Psychology & Psychotherapy, 20,* 107–117. http://dx.doi.org/10.1002/cpp.793

Safran, J. D., & Segal, Z. V. (1990). *Interpersonal process in cognitive therapy.* New York, NY: Basic Books.

Salzberg, S. (1995). *Lovingkindness: The revolutionary art of happiness.* Boston, MA: Shambhala.

Santorelli, S. F., Meleo-Meyers, F., & Koerbel, L. (2017). *Mindfulness-based stress reduction (MBSR) authorized curriculum guide* (Rev. ed.). Shrewsbury, MA: Center for Mindfulness in Medicine, Health Care, and Society, University of Massachusetts Medical School.

Schure, M. B., Simpson, T. L., Martinez, M., Sayre, G., & Kearney, D. J. (2018). Mindfulness-based processes of healing for veterans with post-traumatic stress disorder. *The Journal of Alternative and Complementary Medicine, 24,* 1063–1068. http://dx.doi.org/10.1089/acm.2017.0404

Scott, E. L., Kroenke, K., Wu, J., & Yu, Z. (2016). Beneficial effects of improvement in depression, pain catastrophizing, and anxiety on pain outcomes: A 12-month longitudinal analysis. *The Journal of Pain, 17,* 215–222. http://dx.doi.org/10.1016/j.jpain.2015.10.011

Segal, Z. V., Williams, J. M. G., & Teasdale, J. D. (2013). *Mindfulness-based cognitive therapy for depression* (2nd ed.). New York, NY: Guilford Press.

Serpa, J. G., Taylor, S. L., & Tillisch, K. (2014). Mindfulness-based stress reduction (MBSR) reduces anxiety, depression, and suicidal ideation in veterans. *Medical Care, 52*(Suppl. 5), S19–S24. http://dx.doi.org/10.1097/MLR.0000000000000202

Shapiro, S. L., Carlson, L. E., Astin, J. A., & Freedman, B. (2006). Mechanisms of mindfulness. *Journal of Clinical Psychology, 62,* 373–386. http://dx.doi.org/10.1002/jclp.20237

Shea, T., & Schnurr, P. (2017). *Present-centered therapy* [VA PTSD Consultation Lecture Series: PowerPoint presentation]. Retrieved January 18, 2019, from https://www.ptsd.va.gov/professional/consult/2017lecture_archive/12202017_lecture_slides.pdf

Siegel, D. J. (2007). *The mindful brain: Reflection and attunement in the cultivation of well-being*. New York, NY: Norton.

Siegel, R. D. (2015). Mindfulness in the treatment of trauma-related chronic pain. In V. Follette, J. Briere, D. Rozelle, J. W. Hopper, & D. I. Rome (Eds.), *Mindfulness-oriented interventions for trauma* (pp. 15–18). New York, NY: Guilford Press.

Simpson, T. L., Rise, P., Browne, K. C., Lehavot, K., & Kaysen, D. (2019). Clinical presentations, social functioning, and treatment receipt among individuals with comorbid life-time PTSD and alcohol use disorders versus drug use disorders: Findings from NESARC-III. *Addiction*. Advance online publication. http://dx.doi.org/10.1111/add.14565

Simpson, T. L., Stappenbeck, C. A., Luterek, J. A., Lehavot, K., & Kaysen, D. L. (2014). Drinking motives moderate daily relationships between PTSD symptoms and alcohol use. *Journal of Abnormal Psychology, 123,* 237–247. http://dx.doi.org/10.1037/a0035193

Sinha, R. (2007). The role of stress in addiction relapse. *Current Psychiatry Reports, 9,* 388–395. http://dx.doi.org/10.1007/s11920-007-0050-6

Sipe, W. E. B., & Eisendrath, S. J. (2012). Mindfulness-based cognitive therapy: Theory and practice. *The Canadian Journal of Psychiatry, 57,* 63–69. http://dx.doi.org/10.1177/070674371205700202

Skelly, A. C., Chou, R., Dettori, J. R., Turner, J. A., Friedly, J. L., Rundell, S. D., . . . Ferguson, A. J. R. (2018). *Noninvasive nonpharmacological treatment for chronic pain: A systematic review* (Comparative Effectiveness Review No. 209). Rockville, MD: U.S. Department of Health and Human Services, Agency for Healthcare Research and Quality.

Steenkamp, M. M., Litz, B. T., Hoge, C. W., & Marmar, C. R. (2015). Psychotherapy for military-related PTSD: A review of randomized clinical trials. *JAMA, 314,* 489–500. http://dx.doi.org/10.1001/jama.2015.8370

Stein, M. B., Walker, J. R., Hazen, A. L., & Forde, D. R. (1997). Full and partial posttraumatic stress disorder: Findings from a community survey. *The American Journal of Psychiatry, 154,* 1114–1119. http://dx.doi.org/10.1176/ajp.154.8.1114

Steinert, C., Hofmann, M., Leichsenring, F., & Kruse, J. (2015). The course of PTSD in naturalistic long-term studies: High variability of outcomes. A systematic review. *Nordic Journal of Psychiatry, 69,* 483–496. http://dx.doi.org/10.3109/08039488.2015.1005023

Stephenson, K. R., Simpson, T. L., Martinez, M. E., & Kearney, D. J. (2016). Changes in mindfulness and posttraumatic stress disorder symptoms among veterans enrolled in mindfulness-based stress reduction. *Journal of Clinical Psychology, 73,* 201–217. http://dx.doi.org/10.1002/jclp.22323

Teasdale, J. D., & Chaskalson, M. (2011a). How does mindfulness transform suffering? I: The nature and origins of *dukkha*. *Contemporary Buddhism, 12*, 89–102. http://dx.doi.org/10.1080/14639947.2011.564824

Teasdale, J. D., & Chaskalson, M. (2011b). How does mindfulness transform suffering? II: The transformation of *dukkha*. *Contemporary Buddhism, 12*, 103–124. http://dx.doi.org/10.1080/14639947.2011.564826

Teasdale, J. D., Moore, R. G., Hayhurst, H., Pope, M., Williams, S., & Segal, Z. V. (2002). Metacognitive awareness and prevention of relapse in depression: Empirical evidence. *Journal of Consulting and Clinical Psychology, 70*, 275–287. http://dx.doi.org/10.1037/0022-006X.70.2.275

Teasdale, J. D., Segal, Z. V., & Williams, J. M. G. (2003). Mindfulness training and problem formulation. *Clinical Psychology Science and Practice, 10*, 157–160. http://dx.doi.org/10.1093/clipsy.bpg017

Thakur, E. R., Shapiro, J., Chan, J., Lumley, M. A., Cully, J. A., Bradford, A., & El-Serag, H. B. (2018). A systematic review of the effectiveness of psychological treatments for IBS in gastroenterology settings: Promising but in need of further study. *Digestive Diseases and Sciences, 63*, 2189–2201. Advance online publication. http://dx.doi.org/10.1007/s10620-018-5095-3

Thera, N. (1994). *The practice of loving-kindness (metta) as taught by the Buddha in the Pali Canon*. Retrieved from https://www.accesstoinsight.org/lib/authors/nanamoli/wheel007.html

Treleaven, D. A. (2018). *Trauma-sensitive mindfulness: Practices for safe and transformative healing*. New York, NY: Norton.

Tuerk, P. W., Yoder, M., Grubaugh, A., Myrick, H., Hamner, M., & Acierno, R. (2011). Prolonged exposure therapy for combat-related posttraumatic stress disorder: An examination of treatment effectiveness for veterans of the wars in Afghanistan and Iraq. *Journal of Anxiety Disorders, 25*, 397–403. http://dx.doi.org/10.1016/j.janxdis.2010.11.002

U.S. Department of Veterans Affairs. (2016). *VA/DoD clinical practice guidelines: Management of major depressive disorder (MDD)*. Retrieved from https://www.healthquality.va.gov/guidelines/MH/mdd/

U.S. Department of Veterans Affairs. (2017). *VA/DoD clinical practice guidelines: Management of posttraumatic stress disorder and acute stress reaction*. Retrieved from https://www.healthquality.va.gov/guidelines/MH/ptsd/

Van Dam, N. T., van Vugt, M. K., Vago, D. R., Schmalzl, L., Saron, C. D., Olendzki, A., . . . Meyer, D. E. (2018). Mind the hype: A critical evaluation and prescriptive agenda for research on mindfulness and meditation. *Perspectives on Psychological Science, 13*, 36–61. http://dx.doi.org/10.1177/1745691617709589

van der Velden, A. M., Kuyken, W., Wattar, U., Crane, C., Pallesen, K. J., Dahlgaard, J., . . . Piet, J. (2015). A systematic review of mechanisms of change in mindfulness-based cognitive therapy in the treatment of recurrent major depressive disorder. *Clinical Psychology Review, 37*, 26–39. http://dx.doi.org/10.1016/j.cpr.2015.02.001

van Minnen, A., Harned, M. S., Zoellner, L., & Mills, K. (2012). Examining potential contraindications for prolonged exposure therapy for PTSD. *European Journal of Psychotraumatology, 3*, 18805. Advance online publication. http://dx.doi.org/10.3402/ejpt.v3i0.18805

Van Oudenhove, L., Levy, R. L., Crowell, M. D., Drossman, D. A., Halpert, A. D., Keefer, L., . . . Naliboff, B. D. (2016). Biopsychosocial aspects of functional gastrointestinal disorders: How central and environmental processes contribute to the development and expression of functional gastrointestinal disorders. *Gastroenterology, 150*, 1355–1367. http://dx.doi.org/10.1053/j.gastro.2016.02.027

Veehof, M. M., Oskam, M. J., Schreurs, K. M. G., & Bohlmeijer, E. T. (2011). Acceptance-based interventions for the treatment of chronic pain: A systematic review and meta-analysis. *Pain, 152*, 533–542. http://dx.doi.org/10.1016/j.pain.2010.11.002

Viana, A. G., Paulus, D. J., Garza, M., Lemaire, C., Bakhshaie, J., Cardoso, J. B., . . . Zvolensky, M. J. (2017). Rumination and PTSD symptoms among trauma-exposed Latinos in primary care: Is mindful attention helpful? *Psychiatry Research, 258*, 244–249. http://dx.doi.org/10.1016/j.psychres.2017.08.042

Vlaeyen, J. W. S., & Linton, S. J. (2000). Fear-avoidance and its consequences in chronic musculoskeletal pain: A state of the art. *Pain, 85*, 317–332. http://dx.doi.org/10.1016/S0304-3959(99)00242-0

Vujanovic, A. A., Niles, B., Pietrefesa, A., Schmertz, S. K., & Potter, C. M. (2013). Mindfulness in the treatment of posttraumatic stress disorder among military veterans. *Spirituality in Clinical Practice, 1*(S), 15–25. http://dx.doi.org/10.1037/2326-4500.1.S.15

Wahbeh, H., Lu, M., & Oken, B. (2011). Mindful awareness and non-judging in relation to posttraumatic stress disorder symptoms. *Mindfulness, 2*, 219–227. http://dx.doi.org/10.1007/s12671-011-0064-3

Wampold, B. E., & Imel, Z. E. (2015). *The great psychotherapy debate: The evidence for what makes psychotherapy work*. New York, NY: Routledge. http://dx.doi.org/10.4324/9780203582015

Wang, P. S., Lane, M., Olfson, M., Pincus, H. A., Wells, K. B., & Kessler, R. C. (2005). Twelve-month use of mental health services in the United States: Results from the National Comorbidity Survey Replication. *Archives of General Psychiatry, 62*, 629–640. http://dx.doi.org/10.1001/archpsyc.62.6.629

Watts, B. V., Schnurr, P. P., Mayo, L., Young-Xu, Y., Weeks, W. B., & Friedman, M. J. (2013). Meta-analysis of the efficacy of treatments for posttraumatic stress disorder. *The Journal of Clinical Psychiatry, 74*, e541–e550. http://dx.doi.org/10.4088/JCP.12r08225

Weathers, F. W., Keane, T. M., & Davidson, J. R. (2001). Clinician-administered PTSD scale: A review of the first ten years of research. *Depression and Anxiety, 13*, 132–156. http://dx.doi.org/10.1002/da.1029

Weathers, F. W., Litz, B. T., Herman, D. S., Huska, J. A., & Keane, T. M. (1993). *The PTSD Checklist (PCL): Reliability, validity, and diagnostic utility*. Paper presented at the 9th Annual Meeting of the International Society for Traumatic Stress Studies, San Antonio, TX.

Wessely, S., Nimnuan, C., & Sharpe, M. (1999). Functional somatic syndromes: One or many? *The Lancet, 354,* 936–939. http://dx.doi.org/10.1016/S0140-6736(98)08320-2

Williams, J. M. G. (2008). Mindfulness, depression and modes of mind. *Cognitive Therapy and Research, 32,* 721–733. http://dx.doi.org/10.1007/s10608-008-9204-z

Williams, J. M. G., & Barnhofer, T. (2015). Mindfulness-based cognitive therapy for chronic depression and trauma. In V. M. Follette, J. Briere, D. Rozelle, J. W. Hopper, & D. I. Rome (Eds.), *Mindfulness-oriented interventions for trauma: Integrating contemplative practices* (pp. 91–101). New York, NY: Guilford Press.

Wolfe, F., Clauw, D. J., Fitzcharles, M.-A., Goldenberg, D. L., Häuser, W., Katz, R. L., . . . Walitt, B. (2016). 2016 Revisions to the 2010/2011 fibromyalgia diagnostic criteria. *Seminars in Arthritis and Rheumatism, 46,* 319–329. http://dx.doi.org/10.1016/j.semarthrit.2016.08.012

Index

N

National Comorbidity Survey, 16
National Comorbidity Survey Replication
    study, 16
National Health Service (NHS), 51, 52
Negative alterations in cognitions
    and mood cluster (PTSD
    symptoms), 15
Niles, B. L., 28, 33
Nonjudgment, attitude of, 6, 7, 18, 95
Nonreactivity, 22, 24, 113
Nonstriving, 18
Non-trauma-focused therapies, 17–18

O

Openness, in MBIs, 6, 9, 60
Orientation session, 72–73
Overgeneralized autobiographical
    memory, 44–45

P

Pain, patients with. *See also* Chronic pain
    body scan for, 95–96
    and depression, 41
    loving-kindness meditation for, 105,
        107
    psychoeducation for, 90–91
    sitting meditation for, 99
Pain catastrophizing, 58–60
Pain syndromes, 57
Palmer, Parker J., 74
Parenting, 20
Participation (in group-based MBIs)
    facilitation of, 81–82
    guidelines for, 73, 74
    opting in, 84–85
Patience, 18
Patient-centered, patient-driven care
    model, 70–71
PCL (PTSD checklist), 31
PCT. *See* Present-centered therapy
PE. *See* Prolonged exposure therapy
Peer support, for facilitators, 116
Physical health, of people with PTSD, 6,
    15–16, 40
Physical limitations, individuals with, 41,
    100–102
Piet, J., 49–50

Polusny, M. A., 28, 30–32, 34, 48, 63
Posttrauma sequelae. *See* Trauma-related
    issues
Posttraumatic stress disorder (PTSD),
    4–10, 13–37
    body scans for patients with, 93
    breathing meditation for patients with,
        97–98, 100
    challenges of learning mindfulness for
        patients with, 84–88
    comorbidities with, 40–41
    epidemiology of trauma and, 14–16
    loving-kindness meditation for patients
        with, 108
    psychological treatments for, 16–18
    research on MBIs for treatment of, 7–8,
        27–34
    safety of MBIs for treatment of,
        34–36
    subtypes of, 15
    theoretical models of mindfulness and,
        20–27
    types of MBIs for treatment of, 18–20
Presence, 75
    and being mode of mind, 44
    in body scan, 94
    in mindful movement, 102
    and overgeneralized memory, 45
Present-centered therapy (PCT)
    MBET vs., 33–34
    MBSR vs., 28–32
    safety of MBIs vs., 34
    trauma-focused therapies vs., 17–18
Problem-solving focus, 8, 45, 86
Process-oriented groups, 79
Prolonged exposure therapy (PE), 6, 17, 33
Psychoeducation, 33, 90, 112
PTSD. *See* Posttraumatic stress disorder
PTSD checklist (PCL), 31

Q

Qi gong, 101–102
Quality of life issues, 6, 31

R

Reaction patterns
    breathing meditation to interrupt, 97–98
    in loving-kindness meditation, 105–106
    noticing, 76, 80, 85–86, 92

About the Authors

David J. Kearney, MD, is a staff physician at VA Puget Sound Health Care System and a professor of medicine at the University of Washington School of Medicine. He is the founder and director of the Mindfulness-Based Stress Reduction Program at VA Puget Sound Health Care System. His research has studied the influence of mindfulness-based interventions on a broad range of outcomes, including symptoms of posttraumatic stress disorder and depression, quality of life, pain, gastrointestinal symptoms, fatigue, and attention/memory lapses. His work involves clinical trials comparing mindfulness-based interventions with approaches based on cognitive behavior therapy in a population with a high prevalence of trauma. His work has been supported through grants from the VA Office of Research & Development.

Tracy L. Simpson, PhD, is a clinical psychologist at VA Puget Sound Health Care System and a professor of psychiatry and behavioral sciences at the University of Washington School of Medicine. She is a senior faculty member of the VA Puget Sound Center of Excellence in Substance Addiction Treatment and Education. Dr. Simpson has over 20 years of clinical and research experience with trauma and posttrauma sequelae, and has collaborated with Dr. Kearney on various trials evaluating mindfulness-based interventions for posttraumatic stress disorder (PTSD). She has also carried out trials evaluating pharmacologic and behavioral interventions for alcohol use disorders with and without concurrent posttraumatic stress disorder. Her work has been supported by grants from the National Institute on Alcohol Abuse and Alcoholism, the Department of Defense, and the VA Office of Research & Development.